# Fire Department
## Preplan Worksheet

Date: _____

**General Property Information:**

Building #: _____        Address: _____

Response Area #: _____

Business Name: _____        Building Name: _____

Contact in Case of Emergency: _____

Emergency Phone Number: _____

Occupancy Type: _____

Number of People: _____     Day: _____     Night: _____

Ground Access Obstructions: _____

Overhead Obstructions: _____

**General Building Information:**

Interior Stair: (yes/no)        Stairwell Location(s): _____

Enclosed: (yes/no)        Open: (yes/no)        Doors Locked: (yes/no)

Building Size (Length/Width/Stories): _____/_____/_____

Elevators: (yes/no)

Elevator Door Keys Location: _____

Electrical Shutoff Location: _____

Air Conditioning Location: _____

Water Shutoff Location: _____

Gas/Propane Shutoff Location: _____

Knox Box Location: _____

**Fire Protection Systems:**

Sprinkler System: (yes/no)

Area Covered Type System: _____

FDC Location: _____

Standpipe System: (yes/no)                    Location: _____

FDC Location: _____

Fire Alarm System: (yes/no)                    Location: _____

Reset Procedure: _____

Fire Pump: (yes/no)                    Location: _____

Diesel/Electric/Gas: _____

Emergency Generator: (yes/no)                    Location: _____

Shutoff Location: _____

Special Extinguishing Agent: (yes/no)                    Location: _____

Type: _____

**Construction:**

Exterior Walls: _____        Interior Walls: _____

Flooring: _____

Roof Construction: _____

Attic Access Location: _____

Firewall Location: _____

Ventilation Location: _____

Roof Access Location: _____

High Value Property Location: _____        Access: _____

**Water Supply:**

Location: _____

Distance: _____        Main Size: _____        Color: _____

**Figure 2-2** Sample fire department preplan.

*continues*

**Other Information:**

_____
_____
_____

**Hazardous Materials**

| Chemical | Container Type | Container Size | Total Quantity | *ERG* Number | MSDS Location |
|---|---|---|---|---|---|
|  |  |  |  |  |  |
|  |  |  |  |  |  |
|  |  |  |  |  |  |
|  |  |  |  |  |  |

**DRAWING:**

**Figure 2-2** Sample fire department preplan, continued.

---

### Fire Response Box

A fire response box, or "box," is a traditional fire department term for preplanned resource bundling, designating a predetermined number of resources to be automatically assigned on a given type of alarm. For example, a "full box" for a single-family, residential working structure fire may include two engines, one ladder truck, one rescue squad, one ambulance, and one battalion chief or other supervisor. A box for a commercial fire alarm might include the above resources for a residence plus two additional engines and an additional ladder truck. A box for a high-rise incident might add additional ladders, supervisors, and air support units.

request the equipment through future budgeting processes or to research other solutions to having the equipment available such as mutual aid agreements. Mutual aid agreements are a mechanism through which neighboring or regional jurisdictions can request assistance for a variety of needs, such as additional equipment or staffing for particular incidents.

As departments gather and refine fire plans for specific facilities and occupancies, the plans can be included in the department's master strategic plan to drive departmental growth and may be instrumental in the community's overall growth and sustainment plan.

## Identification of Hazards

In conducting fire preplan assessments, it is important for firefighters to know what hazards, both real and potential, are present in a facility before responding to a call for the particular location. Hazards include permanent or mobile material, practices by the occupants in and around a facility, or anything else that may cause damage or injury. Knowing about hazards is not enough; it is important to know how these hazards might impede operations such as response, rescue, fire suppression, or evacuation, and to what degree these issues must be taken into account.

When identifying hazards, a list of all potential hazards must be made, regardless of the probable impact these hazards have by themselves. In this way, the potential synergy or combinations of the hazards can be accurately calculated, and a risk stratification can be completed. Risk stratification involves determining the danger potential of all identified hazards, the degree to which that hazard is present (eg, quantity of a hazardous substance), as well as any direct or indirect potential consequences of an individual or combination of hazards. In taking an all-hazards approach to preplanning, the following simple and direct questions must be answered:

- What hazards are present? Are there chemicals? Are there confined spaces in the given location? Are these hazards located in particular areas or throughout the entire facility?

How many of these hazards exist, or how much is present?

- How are the hazards detected? Are the hazards detected by electronic alarms or are they undetectable except by specific measuring or detection devices such as carbon monoxide (CO)?
- How can the specific hazards be mitigated or handled? Does the hazard require special protective equipment such as a chemical protective suit versus traditional firefighting bunker gear or does the substance have to be cooled to decrease the vapors from becoming flammable?
- Do these hazards have the potential to increase their effect if they come in contact with fire, water, or other hazards located on the premise (see **Figure 2-3**)?

## Basic Preplanning Concepts

Those responders who would be first on scene should be the persons that go out to see the site and make an initial plan for the most probable potential incident types. The process of identifying hazards with a basic knowledge of the facility permits the crews to know how they would approach the facility if an incident was to occur. It is sometimes more difficult to evaluate an emergency response plan simply by reading the paperwork. Allowing front-line responders to see a space prior to an incident will make them more likely to understand and relate to the drawings and diagrams included in the preplan. In addition to knowing more about the location and the potential or real hazards present, the plan can also be useful in identifying shortfalls in doctrine, tactics, personnel staffing, and availability of appropriate equipment. Preplanning is based upon five basic principles: A preplan must be Comprehensive, Logical, Efficient, and Adaptive, and it should delegate Responsibility (CLEAR).

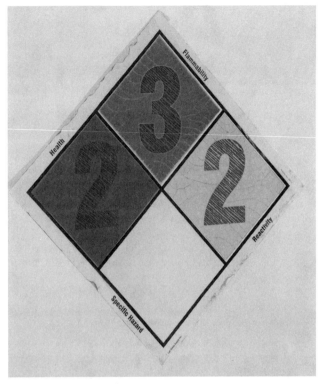

**Figure 2-3** The National Fire Protection Association (NFPA) 704 placard identifies special instructions on what may cause the substance to react violently or present a specific life hazard in a fixed facility.

### Comprehensive

In order for a preplan to be comprehensive, emergency medical service (EMS) agencies must examine all of the factors or issues that may affect the response. These influences may be internal (from within the agency or its operational procedure) or external (the result of emergency incident conditions). A multitude of issues may potentially affect a particular facility. They can be categorized in five major groupings: physical location, hazards, mitigating factors, response, and safety.

Physical location refers to issues such as building construction and layout, routes of access and egress, obstacles surrounding the facility, or hazards inside.

As was mentioned earlier, hazards are any factors that may cause harm or injury. In terms of preplanning, hazard assessment not only includes identifying the individual hazard but also finding information regarding the particular hazard, such as in a material safety data sheet (MSDS). An MSDS is a form, provided by manufacturers and compounders (blenders) of chemicals, containing information about chemical composition, physical and chemical properties, health and safety hazards, emergency response, and waste disposal of the material. EMS must consider how the hazard may affect people, by identifying potential symptoms and treatments (eg, chemical antidotes).

## Material Safety Data Sheet

The MSDS is the vehicle by which employers provide information to employees about hazardous materials and chemicals in the workplace. Occupational Safety and Health Administration (OSHA) Form 174 is the recommended format used to comply with OSHA's Hazard Communication Standard. Chemical distributors are required to provide the MSDS to customers when chemicals are purchased. MSDSs must be readily available in the workplace and must also be accessible to the public if requested. Minimum contents for an MSDS include:

- Name of the chemical (same as is on the container label)
- Chemical and common names of the substance
- List of ingredients
- Statement of the ingredients that are known carcinogens or present other known hazards
- Any specific hazards

In addition to the chemical distributor who provides the product, MSDSs may be obtained for free from multiple sources including many chemical manufacturers, colleges, and universities. The Centers for Disease Control's National Institute for Occupational Safety and Health (NIOSH) maintains a comprehensive Web page devoted to chemical safety issues at www.cdc.gov/NIOSH.

Mitigating factors include information on how to contain, eliminate, or control hazards. These factors may be as simple as large volumes of water to specialized equipment or technical mitigation teams, such as hazardous materials teams.

Response includes everything from special dispatch instructions that may be needed with the initial response, predetermined staging areas, operational issues such as different tactics needed, to overall operations. Regardless of what individual tactic is used, tactics come from two major types: defensive or offensive. In defensive tactics, the majority of efforts are accomplished from the outside of the building; no one initially enters the facility. Defensive tactics are used when it is unsafe to enter the building. In offensive tactics, teams enter the building to find the problem. Many incidents implement a combination of defensive and offensive tactics.

Safety involves issues or tasks undertaken for the safety of responders and civilians alike. Common safety measures include establishing two-person teams so that no one person is alone; if a responder becomes injured, someone is around who can help. Another safety issue is proper personal protective equipment (PPE) for the incident (see **Figure 2-4**). In some types of responses, the typical firefighting PPE can melt or allow toxic materials inside and therefore should not be used.

## Logical

Logical aspects of the plan relate to ensuring the plan is organized in a logical manner so that further response

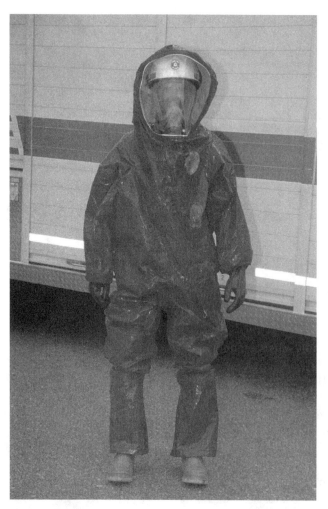

**Figure 2-4** Preplans should incorporate safety measures, such as PPE, to ensure responder safety during incident response.

actions can be anticipated and that the information is able to be understood. This is important in training and administrative issues as well as operational tasks.

### Efficient

Being efficient is tied in with the logical aspect but goes further, because being efficient involves designing processes that identify and plan for the best utilization of all assets. Assets may include people, vehicles, supplies, or administrative tools such as directives, standard operating procedures (SOPs), and standard operating guidelines (SOGs).

### Adaptive

To be adaptive, a preplan needs to be flexible enough to adapt to changing conditions, technologies, or policy. Examples include incorporating the addition of capnography for patient monitoring or the recent addition of a hyperbaric medicine chamber at the closest trauma center. With this additional resource, the treatment and transportation portion of the plan may be modified to enhance patient survival.

### Responsibility

A major aspect of preplanning is the development of responsibility resulting in accountability for response tasks. Responsibility is affixed to specific tasks or issues, to ensure that a specific person is identified and accountable to complete each task. This ensures that important tasks are completed, rather than are assumed to have been accomplished. It also eliminates any confusion about who is designated to complete a certain task.

## Additional Benefits of Preplanning

In addition to the benefits discussed in prior sections, preplanning allows common elements to be identified and used as templates for similar types of responses. The practice of stocking similar resources for similar types of responses is called response packaging or resource bundling. Take for example a motor vehicle crash response: Because most car crashes have common elements and are similar to each other, EMS dispatch and response can be initially similar in terms of the amount of engines, ambulances, and staffing sent to the incident. Preplanning allows for that method of response modeling for comparable incidents and events.

Another benefit of preplanning is that it allows preorganized tactics and modified strategies based on a given facility. EMS agencies are given the opportunity to take into account unique characteristics about the facility. A unique characteristic might be something as simple as an industrial facility that is backed up against a creek or river, prohibiting access from the rear. EMS can take this information into account and modify the preplan based on the specific facility's structure or layout. In other words, the plan allows adaptability in response to changes or to unique features or factors, all the while taking into account the normal or appropriate response package for a specific facility or structure. This practice of utilizing the normal response as a basis for the plan is a key element in preplan development. It is most efficient to base actions on normal practices as much as possible.

In discussing the use of normal response elements in preplanning, it is also important to understand that although a general template can be used, it is essential to mitigate local hazards based on local resources and doctrine. As a result, application of a general, nationwide preplan is usually not appropriate.

An additional benefit of preplanning is the potential decrease in the legal liability to departments because the agency will have already examined the building or facility, assessed the hazards, and made a risk-based decision on how best to proceed. Thankfully, this has not been tested in the court system for EMS agencies as of yet. It could be argued that for failure to reasonably plan for a likely incident, an EMS agency may be found negligent because it had not taken all prudent measures to reduce the potential for an adverse incident outcome. Having plans in place lessens the ability of a potential plaintiff to accuse the department of negligence, because the department has already inspected the facility, made plans, and taken the appropriate action. It has been demonstrated in the emergency management field—and logically assumed to carry over into EMS—that it is more legally defensible for EMS agencies to have a basic plan in place based on prior research about a facility or potential incident, along with any modifications, than to not have a plan in place.

An unintentional or at least an underappreciated benefit to preplanning is that it builds rapport and confidence between an EMS organization and other response agencies such as mutual aid departments, law enforcement, public health, and the Environmental Protection Agency (EPA).

The final benefit of preplanning is that it serves as a proactive means of identifying potential training needs for individual EMS agencies. Certain types of training may be mandated by a regulation or law, or they may be designed, discovered, or developed by individual agencies in response to a particular issue. After an organization's training needs for a response to a particular venue or incident are identified, they can be evaluated, and the plan can be modified as needed.

## Room for Improvement

When comparing fire preplans to EMS preplans, there is some overlap in the basic structure. The most significant difference between these preplans, however, is that the fire service preplan is developed with firefighting in mind. Fire service preplanners will concentrate on such details as the number of engines needed to lay particular hose lines for attack, ladder trucks needed for ventilation and search, the flow calculation of hundreds of gallons of water, and the water pressure needed to reach the seat of the fire.

In EMS, preplans will focus on the elements of patient care: triage, treatment, and transportation. Even if all of the firefighters are also EMS providers—either paramedics or EMTs—the tasks for which they are dispatched to an incident location are not geared towards treatment and transport of patients, but rather are concerned with fire attack, search, and ventilation. In fire preplans, EMS concerns are cursorily addressed, usually with a single triage area and a note that EMS will take care of triage, treatment, and transportation, while the fire department retains overall control. Although, in most cases, the fire department does retain overall control in accordance with the National Incident Management System (NIMS) for such incidents, the salient point is that fire preplans do not adequately address particular EMS concerns. NIMS is the structure for managing an emergency incident, which may require a response of many different agencies. It is designed to provide efficient and effective management from initial response through recovery.

An example of the limitations of fire preplans is that, in many instances, treatment areas are placed for quick evacuation of the facility, but the ratio of patient caregivers to patients is scant. Consider the following scenario.

## Case Study

Imagine if a nursing home in an EMS agency's primary response area has a wing of approximately 20 ventilator-dependent patients, and they are removed from the facility. Where will the patients be placed, how will they be treated, and how will communications be established and controlled while the patients are transported? Furthermore, how will the patients be ventilated without their medical ventilators in place?

Twenty ventilator-dependent patients will cause a severe taxing of most fire departments in the United States, even some of the largest. Fire preplans will not include specific guidance on how and where to obtain additional ambulances. EMS agencies need to have answers to questions such as the following:

> ### Case Study, continued
>
> What trigger points are required to request additional ambulances? Where will the ambulances come from? These questions are not answered in a fire service preplan. For better or worse, the normal fire department response is to call for more and more ambulances, stripping the immediate surrounding area of ambulance coverage, necessitating even more resources in an emergent nature rather than in a predetermined method. This may solve the problem of an ambulance shortage in the short-term sense, but what about the rest of the daily calls that will still come in? What do the ambulances do once they drop off patients; should they come back to EMS control, return to overall incident staging, or do they go back into overall circulation for other calls?

There is no reason why preplanning to resolve these issues cannot be done concurrently with the fire department personnel. It is a more efficient approach, however, for EMS agencies to use their skills and experience to attend to the particulars of EMS issues through preplanning.

# Other Planning Models

The fire department preplan has been explored as a basis for EMS preincident preparation, but there are other planning models that merit consideration as well. These other models include community emergency response plans (CERPs), industrial response plans, the National Earthquake Hazards Reduction Program (NEHRP), bioterrorism response plans (BRPs), and military patrol or operations orders. Although these preplans are different from one another, they have common elements that are instructive in designing EMS preplans.

## Community Emergency Response Plans

CERPs are developed by the emergency management departments (emergency operations centers) and tend to be over 100 pages in length as a complete work, including annexes. These are state and local jurisdictional plans that look at the overall community response—sometimes termed "global response." They usually factor in additional aspects of the disaster paradigm: preparation, mitigation, and recovery.

These plans address EMS in the overall or global perspective, not by covering specific issues, much like national plans do. EMS must be aware of CERPs, because they usually spell out major goals of the overall community response with specific responsibility addressed for the big sections of the plans. These plans are usually designed by emergency managers and not EMS professionals. As a result, the plans may assume or anticipate specific techniques or guidance from EMS. They assume the functions of transportation and patient care will be carried out, in many cases just as they are done under normal circumstances. They do not thoroughly consider the difficulties and extenuating factors involved with transportation from a large event.

## Industrial Response Plans

Industrial response plans are plans designed to address specific industrial sites and are usually required by the Occupational Safety and Health Administration (OSHA) or other regulatory agencies (see **Figure 2-5**). OSHA is the US federal agency that regulates worker safety and, in some cases, responder safety. It is a part of the US Department of Labor. Facilities must have some plan or process identified for worker safety. A key point with regard to industrial response plans is that there are as many different types of these plans as there are industries in the United States. Common industries that have industrial response preplans are petroleum manufacture/transportation/storage facilities, other types of manufacturing plants (particularly where potentially hazardous materials are utilized or stored), and transportation hubs such as rail heads or airports.

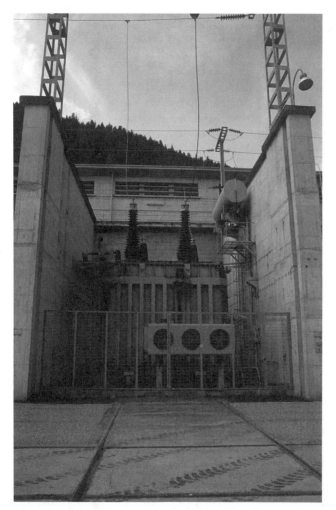

**Figure 2-5** Industrial response plans are designed to address specific industrial sites, such as the transformer station pictured, and are usually required by OSHA.

Many times these plans are designed by engineers who have designed the facility or are developed by business management persons who are not familiar with emergency response operations. This is changing in some industries, as more risk management or safety personnel are learning to be cognizant of how their plans must have some sort of coordination with emergency responders (most likely the fire department). Many still only have a cursory understanding of EMS functions, however, or merely assume that EMS will handle the injured persons as they normally do.

The most common aspects of industrial response plans deal with recognition and detection of an incident, a designated response, and specific industry focus, such as reducing or stopping a leak of petroleum, safety considerations, and integration of public safety assets. Another large component of industrial response plans is the continuity of operations or COOP. This aspect of the plan is designed to detail the extent to which a facility can address various contingencies while remaining operational. Taken to the extreme, the COOP explains how the company will stay in business if an incident occurs.

A significant limitation of the industrial response plan is that, in many instances, the plan is developed without any or significant input from any public safety agency, let alone EMS. As a result, its creators may have made false assumptions in the preparation of their plan. Additionally, these plans are more specifically designed to assist the company than to assist EMS and so may be of limited use to emergency care providers.

The industrial response plan is a good starting point for EMS. Agencies should remember to ask to see the plan when the process of EMS preplanning for a particular facility begins. It is very possible that many hazards and potential complications have already been identified in the industrial response plan. EMS agencies can use this information to their advantage, but must bear in mind the limitations of the industrial response plans.

## National Earthquake Hazards Reduction Program

The NEHRP is a federal program designed to help reduce the hazards of earthquakes and the resulting damage. This program's plans focus on issues such as building construction and other technical aspects of infrastructure. The program is designed to improve inspection of structures and the engineering aspects of buildings to make them more resilient to earthquakes.

## Bioterrorism Response Plans

There are many different plans regarding bioterrorism. Each has its strong and weak points, especially in relation to EMS preplanning needs. Many examine preparedness as a whole health system or only in the context of public health. One method created by B.T. Blythe in 2002, named the "A, E, I, O, U and sometimes Y method" for preparedness for bioterrorism events, is a useful tool for developing EMS preplans for bioterrorism incidents. This six-phase method can be adapted for preplanning in EMS, because it addresses key aspects covering critical areas that must be addressed with any plan:

- *Analysis* of vulnerabilities. This is the process for examining where vulnerabilities exist and how significant the vulnerabilities are.
- *Existing* procedures. Response agencies should research existing protocol for responding to bioterrorism incidents before proceeding with the development of a preplan. Tactics used in these plans may prove useful for guiding the creation of an up-to-date plan taking into consideration current response needs.
- *Identification* of incident prevention measures, both primary and secondary. Primary prevention describes preventative measures taken to avoid the occurrence of an emergency incident, while secondary prevention describes preventative measures taken during an incident to prevent further damage.
- *Organize* a preplanning committee or other functional committees.
- *Utilization* of the plan. Response organizations should work with the response plan to decrease the probability of operational error.
- Scrutinize *yourself* and check on progress. This is done to ensure that an agency is on task and that the plan is relevant.

## Military Patrol or Operations Orders

The next type of plan to examine is the military patrol or operations plan. This is a detailed plan that addresses key components that require attention in order to provide the best opportunity for a successful response. Although these plans do not normally address emergency conditions such as rescue or EMS response, they can be adapted to any circumstance and can serve as a place to begin for EMS preplanning. Operations orders, for example, have been utilized with military response to Hurricanes Andrew and Katrina.

Operations orders are usually orders that come down from higher commands to lower units, while patrol orders are usually at the lower unit level. Whether the plans are operations or patrol orders, the basic format is utilized from the highest to smallest units in the military. As stated earlier, the components of these plans are highly adaptive and easy to use.

The basic patrol or operations order consists of five paragraphs that address the following key aspects: situation, mission, execution, service support, and command and signal. This patrol order is also known as a "five-paragraph patrol order." The individual paragraphs are described in more detail, below:

- *Situation.* This takes into consideration what is happening around the unit, enemy activity, what the weather is like or expected to be, the terrain that the enemy occupies, enemy capabilities—which tells the unit what the enemy can potentially do to them—and finally the enemy's most probable course of action (What does the larger command expect the unit to do based on what they know of enemy tactics and prior behavior?). This paragraph also includes the friendly unit's situations around the particular section, what is happening to the left and right, and who is doing what, especially the higher command.
- *Mission.* This section describes what the unit is expected to do and contribute to the overall plan or strategy. This paragraph outlines the "who, what, when, and where" of the plan.
- *Execution.* This is the "how" of the plan: How will the unit get there? Are there any sub-unit plans that need to be addressed? Are coordination instructions needed to accomplish the mission?
- *Service support.* This is the support or logistics that the unit can expect. This paragraph addresses food, water, ammunition, and anything else that may be needed. It also

addresses transportation to and from the assignment, medical evacuation if needed, and personnel issues such as uniforms or technical equipment.

- *Command and signal.* This outlines communication issues such as primary frequencies, other methods of communication, chain of command from the top to the bottom, and the commander's location throughout the mission.

The patrol order addresses key aspects that EMS preplans will need to address in order to be effective. A comprehensive preplan will permit a safe and effective response to the incident or event.

## A Word on EMS Preplanning Experience

The most important conclusion that has been drawn through emergency services' experience with preplanning is the importance of keeping plans practical, as simple as possible, and readily accessible.

In order for a plan to be practical, it must be realistic in its depth and scope. A practical plan does not assume access to highly advanced technology or immediate assistance. Federal regional resources are not likely to arrive at a disaster site within minutes to a few hours. A practical plan does not assume that all 20 ventilator-dependent patients will be transported from the incident without any complications, within a few minutes, in 20 fully staffed ambulances. Keeping plans "practical" means keeping them grounded in the reality of the organization developing the plan.

Plans must be simple, so that they can be followed in the emergent setting. Plans must be as close as possible in format to the presentation of normal response operations, so as not to confuse those who must implement them. If a plan is similar to those used by crews on a daily basis, and if new information is very simply presented, then a plan has a better chance of working in the field.

"Accessible" simply means having a plan that is not put on a shelf to collect dust, but is rather made available by a chief officer or first arriving response unit for use during an emergency. Personnel should be able to look it up on a computer or have a hard copy inside their apparatus for reference about what they need to accomplish to achieve the goals of the plan. If evacuation is a goal, the plan should inform personnel of where evacuation points are located. It should alert responding units to what is supposed to be going on during the response. It is critical for responders to have this information at their fingertips when they really need it. Whatever the ultimate goal of the plan is, the plan should explain in a realistic and simple manner how to get there. Simply put, a plan left on a bookshelf and not reviewed periodically will be ineffectual and is a waste of resources.

## NIMS, Incident Command System, and Preplanning

Preplanning is not accomplished in a void or just for the sake of doing it. In order to be effective, a preplan must synchronize with the primary and secondary response agencies, as well as the mechanism used to synchronize preplanning efforts with the response agency. That mechanism is the NIMS or the incident command system (ICS).

The ICS is designed to provide a standardized, on-scene, all-hazard approach to incident response preplanning. It was originally designed for wildfire response for large physical areas with a great number of separate responding agencies, many of whom might not know each other much less work together on a regular basis. ICS is based upon a flexible, scalable response that can expand or contract as needed. At an incident scene, responders may be drawn from multiple agencies that do not routinely work together. ICS is designed to give a standardized command and communication format, to optimize operations effectiveness, and reduce the problems and potential for miscommunication at responses to incidents. ICS follows a "first-on-scene" structure, where the first responders at a scene have charge of the scene until the incident has been declared resolved. A superior-ranking responder arriving on scene will seize command, or the incident commander (IC) can appoint another individual to be IC. The IC is in charge of the incident site and is responsible for all decisions relating to the management of the incident.

## ICS Overview

ICS consists of an organizational system that establishes procedures for the management of an overall incident and the mechanism of coordinating personnel, facilities, equipment, and communications. It is a system designed to be used or applied from the time an incident occurs until the need for management and operations no longer exists. ICS is interdisciplinary in the sense that it is useful to fire, police, and rescue responders as well as those with nontraditional response roles as understood by the traditional public safety entities. These additional first response entities include public health and hospital emergency departments.

In the United States, ICS has been tested for three decades of use by emergency and non-emergency responders. All levels of government are required to maintain differing levels of ICS training, and private sector organizations regularly use ICS for management of events. ICS is mandated by law for all hazardous materials responses nationally and for many other emergency operations in most states. The mandate by the Department of Homeland Security (DHS) to use ICS means that in everyday life, virtually all EMS and disaster response agencies have an understanding of the ICS from both a conceptual and working-knowledge standpoint. Furthermore, as part of the National Response Plan (NRP), the system was expanded and integrated into NIMS. The NRP is a federally mandated plan, in which the overall federal response activities are determined, and the responsible federal agencies are identified.

### Incidents and Events

ICS operations are broken up into two areas: incidents and events. Incidents are defined within ICS as unplanned situations necessitating a response. Examples of incidents may include the need for an ambulance (emergent medical situation), hazardous material spills, terrorism, and natural disasters including wildfires, flooding, and earthquakes. Events are defined within ICS as planned situations. Events most frequently necessitate preplanning on the part of emergency responders. Incident command is increasingly applied to events both in emergency management and nonemergency management settings. Examples of events include concerts, parades and other ceremonies, local and state fairs, inaugural activities, and training exercises.

One important component of ICS is that each individual participating in the operation reports to only one supervisor. This eliminates the potential for individuals to receive conflicting orders. This one-supervisor system helps overcome the original difficulties with large-scale incidents by increasing accountability, preventing freelancing, improving information flow, and helping to coordinate operations efforts. The concept of designating a single supervisor to each responder is fundamental to the ICS chain-of-command structure.

### Common Terminology

Another concept brought to light by the ICS is the need for common terminology. Individual response agencies develop EMS and fire protocols separately and sometimes with different uses of terms. For instance, certain East Coast fire services may use the terms "engine," "wagon," or "pumper" to indicate a fire engine that carries water and whose primary use is to pump water. Similarly, EMS agencies may refer to ambulances as "BLS capable" or "ALS capable," although both are ambulances that can transport patients. Additionally, BLS trucks may be referred to as "rescue units," although some systems would consider a "rescue" a truck with hydraulic rescue equipment.

This can lead to confusion, because one word may have a different meaning for each organization involved in a response. These discrepancies must be accounted for during preplanning for multiple-agency responses. When different organizations are required to work together, the use of consistent terminology is an essential element in coordinating group efforts and facilitating efficient communication. The ICS promotes the use of common terminology and has an associated glossary of terms that helps bring consistency to position titles, descriptions of resources and how they can be organized, types and names of incident facilities, and a host of other subjects. The use of common terminology is most evident in the titles of command roles, such as IC, safety officer, or operations section chief.

### Scope of ICS

The incident command structure is organized in such a way as to expand and contract as needed by the incident scope, resources, and hazards. Command is established in a top-down fashion, with the most important and authoritative positions established first. Incident command, for example, should be established by the first-arriving unit. Only positions that are required at the time should be established. For instance, although the role of logistics is a position in the ICS, it is unlikely to be needed in a simple highway motor vehicle accident. In most cases, very few positions will need to be activated. Only in the largest and most complex operations will the full ICS organization be utilized.

### Management by Objective

The next important component of ICS is management by objective. Through this facet of ICS, incidents are managed by working towards specific objectives, ranked by priority. The objectives should be as specific as possible, must be attainable, and must be applicable in larger incidents, if possible, given a working time frame. This same concept can be applied to preplanning: The overall plan can be divided into simple elements with smaller objective plans. These smaller plans can then be added together to develop a comprehensive plan for a major event.

Management by objective can be assisted by limiting the number of responsibilities and resources being handled by any individual. ICS requires that any single person's span of control should be between three and seven, with five being ideal. In other words, one manager should have no more than seven units or people working under them at any given time. If more than seven resources are being managed by an individual, then they are being overloaded, and the command structure needs to be expanded by delegating responsibilities (eg, by defining new sections, divisions, or task forces). If fewer than three, then the position's authority can probably be absorbed by the next highest position in the chain of command.

Additional concepts can assist the goal of management by objective, including incident action plans (IAPs) and comprehensive resource management. An IAP describes the objectives for the overall incident strategy, tactics, risk management, and member safety that are developed by incident command. They are updated throughout the incident and may be verbal or written. Development of an IAP includes measuring strategic operations over a given period of time, known as the operational period. The IAP ensures that everyone is working in concert toward the same goal set for that operational period. The purpose of this plan is to provide all incident supervisory personnel with direction for actions to be implemented during the operational period identified in the plan. IAPs provide a coherent means of communicating the overall incident objectives in the context of both operational and support activities. The consolidated IAP is a very important component of the ICS that reduces freelancing and ensures a coordinated response.

At the simplest level, all IAPs must have four elements:

- *What*? What does an agency want to do? What is the mission? Is it a life safety mission, involving the movement of large numbers of people away from a hurricane or wildfire, or is it an issue of providing healthcare at a papal mass?
- *Who*? Who is responsible for which response tasks? Who will an agency need to coordinate with in order to accomplish the mission?
- *Communication.* How will agencies communicate with each other? How many radio channels will be needed? How many radios will be needed? Is there a primary and secondary method of communication? How will responders communicate up the chain of command, horizontally and laterally?
- *Personnel safety.* What is the procedure if an agency's personnel are injured during operations? Are there any protective measures needed to provide for the safety of the group?

## Comprehensive Resource Management

Comprehensive resource management is another key component of ICS that implies that all assets and personnel are accounted for and can be tracked. This is important both during the event to ensure everyone's safety, but also for potential reimbursement by federal or state disaster agencies or corporate entities that may be required by law to cover part of the event.

Resources exist in various levels of status. Assigned resources are those that are working on a field assignment under the direction of a supervisor. Available resources are those that are ready for deployment, but have not been assigned to a field assignment and may be in a staging location. Out-of-service resources are those that are not in the "available" or "assigned" categories. Resources can be "out-of-service" for a variety of reasons including: resupply after a specific task (most common), shortfall in staffing, personnel taking a rest, or damaged mission essential equipment.

## Communications Planning

Common communications planning is essential for ensuring that responders can communicate with one another during an operation effectively. Equipment, procedures, and systems must operate across jurisdictions seamlessly; this is known as interoperability. Developing an integrated voice and data communications system, including equipment, systems, and protocols, must occur prior to the incident. This is a key step in the preplanning process for an incident type or event (see **Figure 2-6**).

## Responder Roles in ICS

Personnel can ultimately make or break an incident response when all levels of responders understand their roles in the ICS. Members of ICS hold various titles, as follow:

- *Single IC.* Most incidents involve a single IC. In these incidents, a single person commands the incident response and is the final decision-making authority. This position, in some states, is also legally accountable for both the control and accountability for the operation.
- *Unified command.* A unified command is an ICS option that allows representatives from multiple jurisdictions and agencies to share command authority and responsibility, thereby working together as a "joint" incident command team. It will typically include a command representative from the major involved

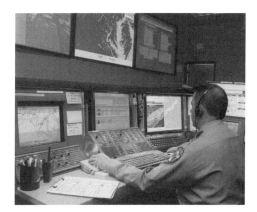

**Figure 2-6** A common communication plan between responding agencies for a major incident or event will ensure an efficient, unified response effort.

agencies and one other member of that group to act as the spokesman, although that person will not be designated as an IC. A unified command acts as a single entity. Unified command may be used in incidents similar to Hurricane Katrina, where numerous state and local agencies were working with the US Coast Guard and Federal Emergency Management Agency.

- *Area command.* During multiple-incident situations, an area command may be established to provide for ICs at separate locations. Generally, one area commander will be assigned, and he or she will operate as a logistical and administrative support.
- *Safety officer.* Members of the command staff will include a safety officer, who will monitor the safety and conditions of operations and personnel while developing measures to account for all assigned personnel.
- *Public information officer (PIO).* The PIO will serve as the conduit for integrated information to internal and external stakeholders, including the media or other organizations seeking information directly from the incident or event. During larger events, a joint information center (JIC) should be developed, providing a means to disseminate information quickly and accurately.
- *Liaison.* This person serves as the primary contact for supporting agencies assisting at an incident.
- *Operations section chief.* Members of the general staff will include the operations section chief, who is tasked with directing all actions to meet the incident objectives. In addition, the planning and logistics section chiefs will serve as support for the operations chief.
- *Planning section chief.* This person is tasked with the collection and display of incident information, particularly as it relates to accomplishing the IAP goals.
- *Logistics section chief.* This person will work in concert with planning to get the materials and resources necessary to carry out the planning section chief's plan for completing the IAP.
- *Finance/administrative section chief.* This person is tasked with tracking incident-related costs, keeping personnel records, monitoring requisitions, and administrating procurement contracts required by logistics.

The ICS within NIMS is based upon preplanning either by type of incidents or for particular events. The NIMS mandate is based on coordination with as many entities as needed to accomplish a mission safely. Preplanning bridges the gap between command systems with response coordination, bringing them together into a cogent method of preparing for an incident before the call for assistance is made.

## Learning From Experience

EMS agencies must recognize that it is possible and beneficial to plan as much as possible for certain contingencies and that, in planning, important issues can be addressed before a crisis begins. Additional benefits of preplanning include being able to view facilities or locations in a systematic and comprehensive manner. Preplanning allows for a rational basis for response action and requires working within the established local and federal legal systems, as well as with other agencies, to coordinate lifesaving efforts.

Additionally, preplans allow for EMS to take conscious, fully thought-out actions in response to particular events and incidents. The fire department's experience with preplanning has shown that the process allows for coordination of multiple issues and goals in order to avoid uncoordinated or conflicting actions by involved responding units. Fire and police departments have different ideas about what needs to occur at an incident or event; preplanning has allowed coordination between these departments to occur prior to an incident response.

Preplans can also serve as a means of implementing policy. If the goal of a city or an agency is to decrease fire deaths, injury in nursing homes, or hospital evacuations, for instance, a carefully developed and clearly presented plan is a means of efficiently implementing policy to accomplish these goals. This is no small benefit; it improves the long-term view of individual departments in higher authorities' eyes.

In static or fluid environments, EMS must realize that the utilization of a plan is effective and that it makes response safer for responders as well as the public. It allows resources to be identified and utilized better than incidents or events attended to without a plan in place. Experience has shown that an effective preplan is practical, simple in concept, and accessible to those who need it.

## Selected References

Blythe BT: *Blindsided*. New York, NY: Penguin Putnam; 2002.

Committee to Identify Innovative Research Needs to Foster Improved Fire Safety in the United States, National Research Council: *Making the Nation Safe from Fire: A Path Forward in Research*. Washington, D.C.: The National Academies Press; 2003.

International City/County Management Association: *Managing Fire and Rescue Services*. Washington, D.C.: ICMA Press; 2002.

Krebs, D: EMS preplanning for large public events. *Fire Eng*; June, 2001.

Pirrallo, RG and Cady, CE: Lessons learned from an emergency medical services fire safety intervention. *Prehosp Emerg Care* 2004;8(2):171–174.

The IEMS National Advisory Committee: Chief executive officer's checklist. *The CEO's Disaster Survival Kit*. Federal Emergency Management Agency and the United States Fire Administration; 1988.

United States Fire Administration: Fire safety lasts a lifetime: A fire safety factsheet for older adults and their caregivers; Emmitsburg, MD: USFA; March, 2006.

United States National Commission on Fire Prevention and Control: *America Burning: The Report of the National Commission on Fire Prevention and Control*; 1973.

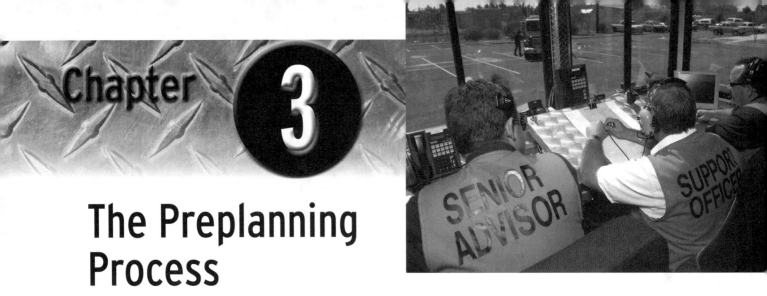

# Chapter 3

# The Preplanning Process

## Beginning the Process

The benefit of planning is that it allows emergency medical services (EMS) agencies to determine the value of different aspects of response to various facilities and incident types. It also places value on the process of examining those facilities, incidents, and response methods. In a way, the process of preplanning is more important than the actual plan. Through examination of the various issues related to individual agencies' responses to various types of facilities and incidents, the planning process allows EMS organizations to assess what is needed for a response, what resources are available, what is not available to the agency, what actions and assumptions are practical, what is not practical, what about the situation is simple, what is complex, what assistance will be needed, and how the EMS agency will get that help.

Preplanning should also begin with a look at coordination or the agency's ability to plan with others. Planning in a vacuum is insufficient at best, and it can lead to complete failure at worst. Incorporating other agencies that may be able to offer direct assistance is absolutely necessary; working with those agencies that only have indirect assistance is also beneficial. Assistance may come from fire departments, public health agencies, environmental agencies, or law enforcement. A multitude of agencies, depending on the needs of the facility, could be involved in the emergency response.

One big question that immediately comes to mind is: How should an EMS agency begin to coordinate with other response agencies? The first step in determining how an agency should coordinate with others is to focus on the facility or event the preplan is being developed for. Then, the EMS agency needs to address the following issues: goal, timeline, need, and partners.

- *Goal.* What is the overall goal of the preplanning effort? Is it to preplan for a facility, such as a nursing home or an industrial site, or is the agency preplanning in preparation for a specific event? Although the basic concepts of preplanning are common among all preplans, it is important to remember that the plan will be implemented at a specific facility or event. A preplanning team must zero in on the specifics of an event or incident before proceeding with the development of a plan.
- *Timeline.* What is the timeline for completion of the plan? Is this a short-term project, or will it take a longer time? EMS agencies must work within a realistic time frame. Establishing a timeline at the beginning of the preplanning process will allow for a more efficient use of time and will keep an agency on schedule.
- *Need.* What is needed to develop an adequate preplan? Agencies should research for other instances of preplanning for similar incidents or events. It is beneficial to look at

what has been done in the past and to assess whether it was effective in terms of outcome. Did the results meet the agency's needs? EMS agencies must also find out what resources are available internally. What in particular is needed (eg, information, equipment) from external organizations (see **Figure 3-1**)? Being thorough and specific in this investigation will lay the foundation for an efficient preplanning effort.

- *Partners.* What partners are needed to accomplish the plan? Who might have the requisite information, equipment, or fit for a specific need?

Once "need" has been determined, and the agency has an idea of who may fill that need, the next step is to figure out how to reach out to those other agencies.

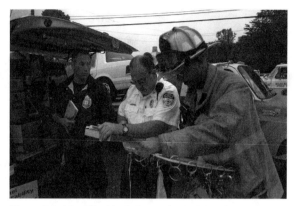

**Figure 3-1** It is critical for EMS agencies to determine what resources are internally available and to decide what assistance (eg, information, equipment, or additional personnel) will be needed to prepare for a successful response.

# Reaching Out to Other Response Agencies

Although there is no guarantee that reaching out will work in every instance, such requests do have a high probability of success when communication is conducted with a genuine attitude of openness, frankness, a willingness to listen, and a desire for mutual benefit. In general, these motivations produce good results when working with others. When outside agencies genuinely ask for assistance, an agency feels good about providing support. For EMS and other responders, the joy of helping others is a natural tenet of their makeup. When in need of assistance, EMS agencies should take advantage of the outside agency's natural need to help, but they should do so with a good attitude.

Some basic issues to consider when reaching out to other organizations include seeking common goals, having a win-win expectation of an outcome, and reaching out to key decision makers within the organization.

## Seeking Common Goals

When considering reaching out, an agency should look for some degree of common ground or need with the agency being contacted for assistance. Is there a common goal of scene safety or effectiveness in patient care? Is there prestige to the organization to be working with the EMS agency? Identifying common goals works to build interpersonal relationships, and it is also an effective tool for guiding preplanning efforts. It allows both organizations to share the tasks, making it easier for both in the long run. It builds trust and fosters thinking from different perspectives, which in turn promotes mutual support for preplanning objectives.

## Ensuring a Win-Win Outcome

EMS organizations should approach the process of working with other agencies with a win-win attitude. An EMS agency should examine what the other organization can provide, while determining ways in which they can assist the other organization and assessing to what extent they will be capable of assisting. The agency may be able to provide training, expertise with other projects, leads on grant opportunities, or outcomes of internal research. It is important that EMS agencies listen to the assisting organization in order to see where both agencies' needs may be met, either directly or indirectly.

### Reaching Out to Key Decision Makers

Reaching out to key decision makers within an organization is an important step when coordinating with an outside agency. Whether the agency's contact with that outside, key decision maker is an equal- or higher-ranking member of the EMS agency, and whether that contact attends the initial meeting or becomes involved later on in the process are not as important as including that decision maker in the preplanning process before too much has been done. The EMS agency heading the preplanning effort should ensure that key decision makers from each organization are aware of what is occurring. Including the key decision makers provides internal limits as well as a champion to request additional resources such as time and personnel.

Once coordination between organizations progresses, the logical question arises of how to incorporate the other organization's plans into the EMS agency plans—how can this be accomplished? Again, it is necessary for an agency to be open, be frank, and listen to how the other agency accomplishes its goals. More importantly, the EMS agency's staff should listen to why the other organization follows certain procedures. Not everything the other organization does needs to be copied by the EMS agency formulating the preplan, as the other organization may have a different mission. If the other organization's procedural "hows" and "whys" do not fit the EMS agency's needs completely, that is alright. The other organization may still have insight that the EMS agency can benefit from.

## Planning With the Goal in Mind

The first step in planning is to determine the goal of the plan. What does the organization want to accomplish? Does the plan support operations, the people who will actually carry out the plan in an emergency? Does the plan need to fit into a regional plan to qualify for federal grants?

An overriding principle behind preplanning is that the plan must make a response safe for the agency's personnel. As such, the plan should inform responders of hazards at specific facilities and events in order to ensure the safety of those responders. This is a simple concept to understand, but may be more difficult to implement. Plans, especially those generated by committees with multiple allegiances, can become complicated. This is usually not due to an individual's or an organization's attempt to derail the plan or the preplanning process, but is probably due to a difference in understanding or familiarity with certain tasks or issues involved in preparing for a particular response. Because of this complicating factor, it is critical to underscore safety in all decisions. EMS agencies should use safety as a common goal to guide preplanning efforts by helping those involved to work through any differences of opinion.

In determining the goal of preplanning, it is essential to make sure that the plan provides direction. Specifically, the plan must direct the individuals or crews who will rely on the plan, now and in the future. Direction involves not only providing the overall intent of the plan, but also the important answers as to what worked in designing the plan, what did not work, and why. This is essential to the goal of the plan because it is likely that the original persons who are familiar with the plan will not be in the same positions they were in when the plan was designed. The intent of the plan and the underlying concerns may not be as obvious later on as at the time the plan was created. The plan may still be valid, but 5 years after the plan was developed (with necessary updates), the effect and direction still need to be evident.

## The Basic Principles of Preplanning

EMS agencies must adhere to three basic principles when formulating preplans: validity, adaptability, and sustainability.

## Validity

In order to be effective, a plan has to be valid. All the assumptions, goals, and expectations of the plan need to be based on reality and based on truly available resources. A plan that assumes access to resources that an EMS agency has no authority over or no ability to access is not a valid plan. It is a mechanism for failure.

In validating the plan, one simple question needs to be continually addressed and answered: Will the plan's expectations and assumptions about what will happen during a response be realistic when the time comes to implement the plan?

The validity of a plan can be based on the research conducted about similar events. EMS agencies may investigate what went right, what went wrong, and the local situation for past, similar responses. Lessons learned by local or federal organizations are particularly helpful in validating a preplan.

## Adaptability

An effective plan will also be adaptable. An EMS agency must address whether the plan can work when it is needed and should make sure key aspects of the plan, such as necessary components of the response and specific equipment, will do what is expected of them. An adaptable plan will not fail for the loss of one element. An EMS agency must examine the high-probability incidents and relevant history and/or data available in order to plan for the failure of key aspects. Because the plan is to be used in the real world and not just as an academic exercise, the actual implementation of the plan should survive certain setbacks. In other words, is the plan a house of cards that will fall if one card is removed, or will it be adaptive, sway, and ultimately stand on its own?

One key element of an adaptable plan is that it focuses on principles instead of practices. This means, when considering tasks or procedures, EMS must decide on what needs to be done to follow the principle. Then, preplanners must design the task or procedure to accomplish the principle rather than any one specific way of accomplishing the task or objective. Consider the example of ventilating a patient: There are multiple ways and techniques to ventilate a patient ranging from endotracheal intubation, King or Combitube insertion, bag-valve ventilation, and supplemental oxygen administration. The major principle of patient ventilation is ensuring the patient can receive and move oxygen in the lungs. The manner or practice is dependent on the local situation of education/training, protocols, and experience. The key is to not to get caught up with a particular practice, but to determine the principle and then design a system to support that principle. A preplan may include multiple suggested practices: primary, secondary, and so on.

Another example in which principle should overrule practice is in the development of a communications system during preplanning. In many after action reports (AARs) from major incidents, disasters, and even trainings, communications (both human systems and actual technology) are often cited as failing or in need of repair. With this in mind, EMS agencies must consider the principle behind communications. The principle is to communicate. In designing the processes or practices that support communication, a primary and secondary means of communication should exist within any adaptable communications plan. EMS should also assess the need for tertiary or more backups with the plan.

## Sustainability

Finally, EMS agencies should create plans that are sustainable. Creating a plan that is only going to last for 2 years requires a great deal of effort but will have very little impact. A plan that can be reviewed and modified as buildings, organizations, resources, technology, and funding change is considered sustainable (see **Figure 3-2**). Sustainability allows the plan to move and grow as everything else does, instead of becoming stagnant and irrelevant.

As technology changes, the plan need not completely change or be scrapped. Perhaps only specific areas of the plan will be affected by changes in technology. These should be modified

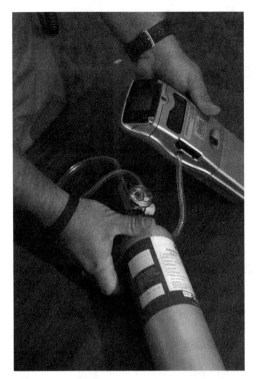

**Figure 3-2** The true test of a preplan's adaptability lies in the ease with which it may be modified to meet changes in technology, buildings, organizations, resources, and funding.

accordingly. The EMS preplanners' goal is to create basic preplan principles that will withstand the test of time. It is unthinkable to use a 1950s civil defense map and technological assumptions to plan for a building built in the twenty-first century. The principles and structure of those plans, however, have very likely informed more modern ones.

## Making Plans Accurate and Accessible

After the goal of the plan is determined, other key issues must be addressed. Is the plan accurate and accessible? In examining whether the plan is accurate, it is necessary to evaluate whether the data or information in the plan is up to date. Consider, as examples, area codes or telephone extensions. It is important also to determine whether the resource information is accurate: Did the reports really demonstrate a fact, or is this someone's opinion? Are these facts based solely on rumor?

A plan should also be accessible to its end users, and they should receive any necessary, new training in preparation for the implementation of the plan. EMS agencies must ask whether the lowest- or highest-ranking person on the scene will be able to look at the plan and see what needs to be done. Where will the plan be housed, and what method of plan retrieval will be used? Is the plan in a binder on all apparatus, is it contained in a PDF document, or is the plan attached and/or linked through the dispatch computer? Have the crews practiced the plan or at least key tasks or objectives?

### "It Can't Happen Here"

What if a 25-year-old EMS responder were asked to remember the flooding in his or her city around 1900 or 1911? What measures were used to control the flooding of the downtown hospital or doctor's office? What about the effects of the Great Influenza of 1918? What did the city do when the flu hit and killed hundreds or thousands of people in a few weeks? Most people cannot remember such events because most were not alive at that time. The lessons learned from those events, in most cases, have been lost.

When it comes to disasters, large events, or other significant incidents, people, public safety organizations, and communities have short memories. Emergency response agencies may remember Hurricanes Katrina and Rita, the San Francisco earthquake of 1989, or the fires in Southern California in 2007, because they lived through that time and those events impacted the way they do what they do, to some degree. People usually remember the press accounts and what happened in their immediate community during an emergency event. They may also remember issues that piqued their interest, such as the responses to disasters, how they developed, the way in which resources were used, and how the events changed or evolved day by day or hour by hour. Those who were affected will remember these events and any important lessons learned. Those who were not directly affected will move on with their lives in a relatively short period of time because they believe it cannot happen again; they believe it will not happen to them. This applies even for those who work in emergency services.

---

**"It Can't Happen Here," continued**

This attitude, often referred to as the "it can't happen here" syndrome, is very common, and it can have a devastatingly negative impact on planning. A community or individual may look at events such as Hurricane Katrina or the San Diego County fires and say "Yes, it happened to the people on the Gulf Coast or California, but it cannot happen to me. I will not have hurricanes or large wildfires." Complacency becomes the status quo; it is accepted and at times even promoted by those in authority using this false logic. This is a dangerous attitude for individuals, but it can be devastating when emergency response organizations share in these false, although comforting, assumptions.

---

## Being Proactive in EMS Preplanning

Generally, when fire departments are in charge of preplanning, their attitudes are not oriented to be proactive in the particulars of EMS. Their focus is fire response. This is natural, as the preplan has to be approved by the station officer and in many instances the duty officer for their district. They are "graded" on what the station officer and duty officer look for: Fire departments must be proactive in terms of determining the need for "x" engines, accomplishing "y" functions at a fire, and directing so many trucks to do "z" at a fire response.

For fireground functions, the EMS role on scene is increasingly a role of rehabilitation and medical screening for firefighter safety. This involves taking blood pressures, monitoring carbon monoxide levels, and providing fluid therapy for rehydration. There is currently a nationwide initiative for "everyone to come home alive" from a fire incident, and not surprisingly, the asset best suited for this function is the EMS crew on scene. Although this is a worthy cause, it should not be the primary purpose or goal for EMS. EMS functions and concerns are not particularly well covered when it comes to preplanning for a fire, as the personnel are biased towards fire response and support of fireground operations.

In non–fire-based EMS agencies, a similar situation exists. If any preplanning takes place, it is usually performed by field personnel who are familiar with the facility or location. They prepare the preplan based on their interaction with the facility and, although the plans developed should have more of a focus on EMS issues, it cannot be assumed. This is not to criticize those EMS personnel involved in the development of such preplans, but it is important to bear in mind that the field personnel will be biased toward their daily tasks and interactions. Their preplans will not be comprehensive, as a result.

## Roadblocks to Preplanning

When an EMS agency first considers the process of preplanning for an incident such as a fire, large gathering, or disaster, the staff must understand that the very mention of the topic may bring out certain attitudes. These attitudes can range from a lack of interest to fervent support. Some responders may ask: "Do we really need to preplan? How will the process benefit us?" Preparing to deal with a potentially resistant environment along with other possible roadblocks that may arise is an important step in propelling preplanning efforts forward. In short, agency leaders should be aware and informed of all the issues surrounding the preplanning process. Apathy, ignorance, "paper plan" syndrome, and minimal federal or state funding are major impediments to any preplanning effort.

### Apathy

EMS must be aware of the potential for apathy or a lack of enthusiasm for the process on the part of responders. There may be several causes for this apathy, including a lack of understanding of

EMS functions and a lack of knowledge about the preplanning process. Regardless of why apathy is present, it is important for agency leadership to take the following approach in dealing with it: Provide an overview of the process, and then begin research on the incident or event.

EMS preplanning leaders should provide an overview of what the agency is expected to accomplish. They should be as specific as necessary, in order to clearly articulate this information to any doubters of the process. It may be helpful to start with a presentation of the overarching preplanning goals, objectives, and an explanation of what will be necessary to successfully respond to a specific type of facility or incident. To help persuade others of the importance of preplanning, it is important to address the benefits of preplanning to the specific agency.

A second tactic for combating apathy is to conscientiously gather data and research information regarding the facility or incident type. This research should indicate what went right or wrong regarding past EMS operations at the particular facility or incident. Beginning the necessary research is a positive action, and it may persuade more people of the need for preplanning by demonstrating that it is possible for the agency to combine efforts to accomplish the task at hand. Actions taken to deal with apathy may persuade some doubters, but may not always meet with unanimous support.

## Ignorance

EMS leaders will also need to address ignorance about the process before proceeding with preplanning. Ignorance goes hand in hand with apathy, but it is not expressed in the same manner. Ignorance is a lack of awareness with regard to something. Ignorance is overcome in the same manner as apathy, but with more of a focus on education about the process. By giving responders the knowledge needed to begin the preplanning process, leaders provide their crews with confidence in the goals and each responder's ability to contribute to the preplanning effort.

### "Someone Else Will Do It"

The "someone else will do it" attitude impedes proper preplanning efforts. Many people, including those in the EMS community, believe that if a significant incident or a disaster occurs, someone else will take charge and that it is not important for EMS to preplan. It is true that someone else such as the fire department or emergency manager may be in charge of the overall incident, because EMS is usually limited to medical care. The stark reality is, however, that EMS responders are that "somebody." Who else but EMS knows the "who, what, when, where, and how" of patient treatment and transport? Leaving the preplanning as the sole purview of the fire department or emergency management may not be the best method or produce the best outcomes for the patients involved.

## "Paper Plan" Syndrome

Many departments and agencies have developed a myriad of plans to direct operations through preplanning or otherwise. EMS agencies will have individual plans on file to meet a specific issue—such as flood, hurricane, or tornado responses—or combination plans that simultaneously address multiple kinds of incidents. In many instances, these plans were not really intended to be utilized; they were designed to meet funding programs. Such plans are known as "paper plans." Paper plans were not developed with the explicit intention of implementation. As a result, the assumptions used during the plans' creation have a high probability of being false or invalid. Although it is still a matter of fiery dispute, it is likely that some plans for New Orleans were paper plans meant to meet the funding needs of different agencies and were not true emergency evacuation or treatment plans for citizens. The development of paper plans poses a significant danger. An incident might occur, and someone who is not privy to the nature of the paper plan will attempt to activate and implement the inadequate plan. This responder might be new to the position or may take the plan more seriously than its authors. Regardless of why the plan is implemented, it has the potential to be followed in a true emergency situation, and it can have disastrous results.

### Federal or State Funding

When looking at government action lists, preplanning for EMS issues usually is not high on that list. Instead, these programs focus on issues such as comprehensive municipal preplanning for disasters. EMS preplanning rarely receives the backing of the higher officials in federal or state government. EMS planning that is not incorporated directly in a large event or key facility planning doesn't have the visibility required to garner the attention necessary to qualify for most national and state-wide initiatives or funding grants.

Over $3 billion have been provided to response agencies through federal grants over the past few years, with over $100 million designated specifically for EMS agencies. The Department of Homeland Security (DHS) provides funds in this order: law enforcement, fire, and then EMS. This allows law enforcement to have money for patrol functions, bomb disposal units, training, canine resources, and communications. Fire departments are considered next for funding, and their priorities include fire apparatus, overtime and training, and hazardous materials issues. Even in fire-based EMS, the percentage of funding is disproportionate to what is reflected in the call volume. According to several large city fire departments, EMS runs account for approximately 75% of their calls, but the funding for EMS is 20% to 25% of the budget. A small remaining portion of the funding is given to non-fire department EMS agencies. In many cases, even when the EMS agencies receive the money, it is needed to address normal training and equipment needs, and does not go directly to the preplanning effort.

Another avenue of funding for some fire-based EMS or individual EMS agencies is the Metropolitan Medical Response System (MMRS), which provides funding, usually through grants, for densely populated cities. This money is bioterrorism-based and comes from the Department of Health and Human Services (HHS) to support response to a bioterrorist event. The money can be used for individual or team training, or towards equipment purchases such as mass-casualty incident trailers and response vehicles. Preplanning as a function of these agencies is not specifically identified and funded as separate aspects but must be rolled into the other portion of the funding.

The last source of funding is the most common: The normal budget through a city, county, or as a business. This money has to be divided between operational costs, training, administrative concerns, and prevention efforts.

Regardless of the source of funding, the effect is the same: Preplanning is often not a high priority. There is no real federal or state champion of funding programs for preplanning. For those personnel who participate in preplanning, it is an additional duty rather than a primary function of the job.

This lack of federal or state funding does not imply that EMS preplanning should not be a high priority. Rather, the message to EMS is that the responsibility is theirs to make a difference in the way they approach treatment and transport during emergency incidents and disasters in their own districts. Preplanning is exactly what should be done because of the lack of federal or state funding; it is overwhelmingly beneficial and does not have to cost a significant amount of money.

## The Need for EMS Preplanning

With the fire department already engaged in preplanning, why is it important for EMS to develop their own preplans? The reality is that the fire department has little training and education or even experience in planning for EMS issues. Most degree programs in the fire service fall into three main areas: public administration, fire science and suppression technology, and business administration.

Public administration covers general areas of municipal administration, budgetary issues, and management theory. Fire science programs are based on theory of response, strategic and tactical considerations, as well as management of fire service personnel. Although this coursework is related to EMS in many aspects, the specific topics of how EMS response differs from fire response and where the lines of control of functions (rescue, triage, and suppression) diverge or converge are focused on the fire side of the equation. Fire science/technology does not adequately address EMS issues in general and specifically in terms of preplanning. Business administration is even further distant from EMS, focusing on business plans, continuity of business operations, strategic planning, productivity, and profit/loss measures. Additionally, emergency management texts do not address EMS issues adequately, as this discipline is not oriented toward a specific function. The combination of a lack of fire texts and curricula that adequately address EMS issues results in a lack of knowledge concerning EMS response needs on the part of fire departments.

College level courses in firefighting aside, even basic firefighting texts do not adequately describe preplanning in any true sense and provide minimal insight into EMS needs. It should be noted, as a result, that fire preplans are severely limited in terms of providing comprehensive overview of EMS' role during a given response.

Fire department preplans can be useful to EMS preplanners as a starting point, but they are woefully inadequate in outlining protocol for coordination with other agencies (other than other fire departments for mutual aid). Staff in a fire department EMS, private EMS, or in third service need more coordination with external agencies and organizations due to the nature of EMS patient care. Coordination in EMS, for example, involves coordination with medical receiving facilities, additional transport services, and possibly integration with public health.

For example, it is simple in a fire plan to say that there is a need to evacuate a certain wing of a hospital. When it comes to EMS, however, there needs to be explicit protocol for what emergency personnel should do to assist a bariatric person on a specialty bed that weighs 1,000 pounds plus the weight of the patient. In this case, it is necessary to understand that to evacuate a bariatric patient without pre-identified methods is difficult at best. It is likely that the 1,000-pound bed and the patient are going to move out 5 feet from the facility door, hit a grass field, and then the bed will bury itself into the ground because the wheels are designed for smooth surfaces only.

Another example of an EMS issue to consider during preplanning is how someone will ventilate a person on a ventilator once the electricity is cut. How long can one person manually ventilate a patient? It requires several people, including backups. These are practical questions that need to be addressed. Most fire plans do not examine these aspects of hospital evacuation or other EMS-related issues in plans for other facilities. For this reason, it is imperative that EMS agencies take it upon themselves to preplan for EMS operations at emergency incidents.

## Case Study

Warren Porter visited several local fire departments to review prefire plans for medical facilities and nursing homes. The plans showed in great detail hydrant locations, and access of parking locations for follow-on vehicles for second and third alarms. They included a lot of specifics concerning fire-related aspects of emergency response, but seemed to have a dearth of information on EMS issues. EMS issues addressed in these plans included how to evacuate large numbers of people, response procedures and priorities, trigger mechanisms for the decision to conduct full evacuation, partial evacuation, or to shelter-in-place.

**Case Study, continued**

In addressing evacuation, for instance, the fire preplan did not seem to know where to relocate residents and/or patients. In several instances, the plans suggested evacuating a nursing home population to an uncovered parking lot. Imagine that mixture of 50 patients and/or residents needing to be evacuated; in addition to the 50 persons present are 20 ventilator patients and 10 Alzheimer's patients. How would these patients fare under the suggested evacuation plan, on a hot summer day or a cold winter night in an open parking lot? What kind of resources would be needed, not only to ventilate patients, but to shelter them from the environment?

EMS agencies must contribute their expertise in patient care and transportation to the preplanning process, as it will prevent ineffective plans from being implemented.

## Coordination

In the preceding section, the term "coordination" with external agencies was used. This is a broad term that needs to be clarified. In order to coordinate, it is first necessary to define the end goal, define intermediate objectives necessary to reach the goal, and then accomplish the tasks associated with this phase of preplanning. Many questions immediately come to mind: Who will an agency coordinate with? What information is needed and from whom will an agency get it? When should coordination take place? In the end, who is in charge or responsible for all of these steps? These questions may appear simple at first glance, but are not as simple as they sound.

Determining who to coordinate with is tied in with what an agency needs to achieve a specific goal, and it will not necessarily be the same with each preplan. Consider the example of developing a preplan to assist a bariatric nursing home patient. In this case, it will be necessary to coordinate with the nursing home to identify, first, whether a bariatric patient resides in the facility. If yes, the agency must research any additional conditions this patient has that may require specific assets in case of a facility evacuation.

For this same example, it is also necessary to work with the fire department for rescue considerations such as staffing needed to safely move the 800-pound patient. It is also necessary to coordinate with any potential receiving hospitals for continued treatment of this patient and to ensure the availability of special beds. This is necessary, because hospitals will have a relatively limited number of bariatric hospital beds available. The EMS agency will also need to ascertain the capability of these receiving facilities to handle any comorbid conditions. It may also be necessary to coordinate with a bariatric transport unit if the local EMS agency does not have that capability.

If the agency does not have the transport capabilities, a plan of action should be developed for assisting the patient until a transport unit arrives. Will the EMS agency need to coordinate with additional patient treatment personnel? Will the bariatric unit be automatically dispatched with the call to that facility? It may be necessary to coordinate with dispatch or communications to verify availability and to request the asset, either at initial dispatch or when other pre-identified aspects of the response have been determined. This will require further coordination with the facility and fire department linked with communications to determine the appropriate triggers for dispatch. That inevitably leads to asking the question: What does the EMS agency want or need to know?

The more that the EMS agency knows about the incident or facility they are planning for, the more they will need to further coordinate. Again, using the bariatric patient as an example, while coordinating with the nursing home on patient types and locations it may be helpful to the preplan to know how many technology-dependent residents live at the facility. How many bariatric patients are currently receiving care at the facility, and what prearranged plans does the facility have to accommodate these patients during an evacuation? Are bariatric patients expected to be transported to one or multiple receiving facilities? In addition, it would be useful for EMS to find out who is responsible for developing and executing the facility's evacuation plan, as well as determining what plans are already in place. EMS agencies should find out who has the plans and the locations of key people or documents.

When coordinating with the fire department, it is useful to know operational procedures such as an average response staff total, what number of fire personnel are EMT or paramedic, and how fire response will be impacted if EMS has to utilize qualified fire personnel for patient care. Furthermore, EMS should question fire inspectors for information on the layout of the facility or other special knowledge that can assist EMS with the preplan.

When coordinating with potential receiving facilities, it may be useful to know such things as how many bariatric and technology-dependent patients they can handle at one time, on a good day or bad day. It may also be helpful to discover any warning communications to the receiving hospitals that allow them to activate their plans in the case of several incoming patients. Arriving with multiple technology-dependent patients can temporarily shut down an emergency room. The hospital may need some lead time to call for additional resources.

The next question that should be asked and addressed is "when should coordination take place?" This question is the easiest to answer, but the answer is more difficult to implement. EMS agencies should begin coordinating as soon as the process of preplanning begins. Coordination should be one of the initial actions taken and should be a continuous process throughout preplanning. The analogy in EMS terms is: When does patient assessment stop? It doesn't; it is an ongoing process until the patient is delivered to the hospital and a proper hand-off has occurred. The same principle applies to scheduling coordination. Coordination is probably the most beneficial action that an agency can perform, and it has benefits well past the basic preplan as evidenced by New Jersey EMS with the US Airways aircraft that landed in the Hudson River in January 2009.

The last question that has to be asked is "who is in charge or responsible for this preplan?" That question has two aspects; the first is "who is overall responsible for an incident?" In many states it will be the fire department that will have overall command at a large incident. That point is legislated from the state. The second aspect of this question is "where does the focus of most EMS preplans interface with other agencies?" It is in this aspect that EMS is responsible for issues surrounding the treatment and transport of patients.

## Use of Technology

Over the last several years there has been a revolution in mobile computer systems and data storage. Data storage that once took bookcases and storage rooms now takes a flash drive in a person's pocket. This revolution has also moved into the public safety arena with the addition of mobile data transponders (MDTs), which are now available in multiple apparatus, including ambulances and fire engines (see **Figure 3-3**). This technology allows the end users, the people who are responding to the incident, to utilize electronically stored and updated plans. Before this revolution, the information had to be paper-based. In many instances, the plan was put on the shelf and never updated.

Technology makes plans more available. Plans can be saved in PDF format, or they can be stored, sorted by multiple databases, and cross-referenced. The goal of making all of these forms of the information available is to make plans accessible in whatever format is available to the responders on the scene. The key message to agencies is simple: A plan that is not accessible by those who need it might as well not have been created.

This does not mean there is no need for paper-based planning, in a binder or notebook, which can still be used as a backup and as a reference. It should be noted that in disaster situations, both local and large scale, one of the recurring issues is failing technology. Again, this may be a pure technological issue or an issue of human interface, which depends upon the scope and depth of responder training.

The two key take-home messages regarding whichever technology application is utilized is, first, that it is necessary for EMS to ensure that those who will need to utilize the preplan have access to the preplan. The second conclusion to be drawn is that EMS agencies must ensure that the preplan has been reviewed by all that may use it, in the format that is expected or planned to be used in the field.

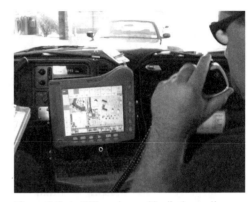

**Figure 3-3** An MDT can be used to display routing information transmitted from the dispatch center.

## General Steps of the Process

General steps of the preplanning process include gathering information, involving coordinating entities in the effort, planning for most incidents in a general sense (using the 80/20 principle), conducting a hazard analysis, and accomplishing a capability analysis.

### Gathering Information

The first general step of preplanning is to gather pertinent information. This research will provide the "who, what, when, where, and how" that are needed to accomplish the response goal. Information gathering can be accomplished by first researching organization documents such as prior plans or events that the agency has been involved in. Another resource could be to use any incidents in the region or state and gather information from the various agencies on what they did, how they did it, what went right, and more importantly what went wrong.

After researching locally or within the state, EMS agencies should look nationally at organizations that have web sites set up to help with first responder organizations. These organizations include the Department of Homeland Security (DHS) Lessons Learned Information Sharing (www.llis.dhs.gov), National Fire Academy, emergency management organizations, and public health schools or organizations such as Yale New Haven Center for Emergency Preparedness and Disaster Response (www.yalenewhavenhealth.org/emergency/index.html) or Johns Hopkins Center for Public Health Preparedness (www.jhsph.edu/preparedness/).

Nongovernment resources exist for EMS as well, such as the peer-reviewed journals that deal with response and disasters, the PUBMED Web site that houses peer-reviewed medical journals and is a great source for topic-related materials, as well as other peer-reviewed journals such as *Prehospital and Disaster Medicine, Crisis Response Journal*, and the *International Journal of Mass Emergencies and Disasters*. Although many of these journals and Web sites are oriented toward disasters and not all preplans are developed for disaster situations, these resources offer a lot of material that can be applied to an EMS agency's general approach to preplanning.

Once data are gathered, the most useful information can be organized and then applied to the plan. It is important to note that not all data gathered will be pertinent to the plan. Some information may be directed at other areas of emergency response and may not be usable as it is not applicable to EMS functions. Although it is beneficial to thoroughly research an event, facility, or incident during preplanning, it also is critical to evaluate the information gathered in terms of the agency's goal in preplanning. The aim is to look at the goal, gather anything that might be relevant, and then ask: Does this relate to the preplanning goal? If so, how?

Preplanners should incorporate any lessons learned from similar facilities, organizations, and even dissimilar entities by looking for similarities and lessons learned on how others have dealt with incidents or utilized their preplans. As an example, one fire department went to a neighboring department when a large nursing home and rehabilitation center was being built in their city.

They inquired about issues of EMS response such as potential staff level changes, response matrix modification (What type of equipment is sent, to where, and for what purpose?), and response impacts. EMS agencies must ask the necessary questions, see what answers are available, and then incorporate their findings into preplan development as best as possible.

## Involving Coordinating Agencies

After gathering the information, it is necessary to begin to develop the plan with those agencies noted in the coordination section. This should include any additional partners who have been identified in the information-gathering phase and are able to assist. As mentioned earlier, these partners may be other EMS agencies, public health, or any other interested or involved entities. These entities may be assisting voluntarily or involuntarily, depending on the goal of the plan, the facility or venue the plan is designed to address, as well as who mandated the plan. If the plan is to address a large mass gathering with the state governor, for example, then other agencies such as the police and public recreation and parks may be required to assist.

## The 80/20 Principle

In preplanning, it is impossible to plan for every eventuality. The 80/20 principle was developed to address the inability to plan for all possibilities. The goal of preplanning should be to plan for most incidents in a general sense, since approximately 80% of incidents have common aspects such as response, command, and logistics. It is important to examine the 80% commonality with standard procedure and the 20% deviation from the norm.

First, 80% of hazards can be covered with a comprehensive plan that is based on normal operational activities. This is an important aspect that cannot be overlooked. People will be able to follow what they normally do; if a plan accounts for this with only a small deviation from standard operations, then the execution will be easier and safer. In essence, the more an individual aspect of the plan is practiced, the better it will work; the less a procedure strays from the norm, the safer it will be to implement.

The other 20% applies to special incidents. These are incidents that have a relatively significant difference from the normal type of incident. They have a firm basis in the 80%, but must be modified because of some special or unique aspect. Examples of unique aspects may include the amount of resources needed to mitigate a hazard, which could relate to access to the facility, or the need for specialized equipment not typically utilized in response.

The relationship between the 80% commonality and 20% deviation from standard procedure may be seen in this example: A particular EMS agency routinely plans for mass gatherings of 300 or 400 people, for a football game or rally in their community. Staff and ambulances are tasked to support the event and then pre-positioned to assist 400 people. EMS has recently been tasked, however, to medically support a political event coming into town and it is expected to attract a crowd of 50 thousand people. There is a significant difference between responding to a mass gathering of 50 thousand and one of 300 people, but the basic premise is maintained. The agency must plan for a mass gathering, as usual, but tailor their response planning for the event's unique aspect of a crowd of 50 thousand people. The unique needs of this event will certainly include additional ambulances and staff. Other issues that may be significant, however, include a more complex communication method and updated procedures. Such issues will include ensuring access and egress for transport units, provision of additional roving or medical treatment tent staff and supplies, coordinating for increased law enforcement presence, as well as preparing a greater cache of medical supplies and protective gear.

### Preplanning Practices

**The 80/20 Rule**

The 80/20 rule suggests that 80% of hazards associated with an event, facility, or potential incident can be covered with a comprehensive plan that is based on normal operational activities.

## Hazard Analysis

When looking at the hazards, it is necessary to systematically gather information about the facility, event, or incident, in order to have a full understanding of what could happen. EMS agencies must ask what is possible and what is probable at a given facility, incident, or event. This assessment is called risk or hazard analysis.

Depending on the facility, event, or incident being planned for, thousands of emergency conditions are possible. EMS should examine not just what is possible but also what is probable. Hurricanes along the Atlantic coast or typhoons on any coast of the country are possible and, obviously, probable. Would the same be said, however, for the interior of the country in Denver, CO or Salt Lake City, UT? Though hurricanes and typhoons are possible in these regions, they are not probable. To determine whether something is probable versus just possible, EMS agencies should look at the history of what has happened in a given region or similar regions in the country. Then, they should look at the number of times a particular incident has occurred and how many years passed between the occurrences. The more frequently an incident has occurred in the past, the higher probability exists that such an event will occur again. Some will say that because a flipped coin has the same probability at any given toss to reveal "heads" or "tails," it is also impossible to plan the probability of an event. Though the outcomes of coin-tosses are somewhat arbitrary, this is not the case for physical events. Factors other than chance influence the probability that an emergency incident will occur at a given facility or event.

During preplanning, EMS should examine those aspects in the plan that are probable, take the top three or five, identify the hazards associated with those incidents, and examine the probability that those hazards could impact the EMS agency. In looking at probabilities, an EMS agency must understand the realities of certain events. During Hurricanes Katrina and Rita, certain inland areas did not experience an actual hurricane, but other surrounding states might have been impacted by tornados that are spun from hurricanes. This example shows that, in certain instances, it may be necessary for EMS to plan for secondary events that stem from locally improbable incidents.

Hazard assessment should evaluate all potential hazards within a structure or facility and determine what impact those hazards will have on the plan, in terms of responder and patient safety. There are a number of things to consider when analyzing hazards:

- What hazards are there?
- Where are they?
- How much (quantity) or how many are there?
- How are the hazards detected? Are the hazards detected by sound alarms, or are they undetectable without the use of certain measuring devices?
- How can the specific hazards be mitigated?

Once the hazards are identified, whether there is one or 100, EMS must plan for effective mitigation of each hazard. If a certain hazard cannot be mitigated, EMS must determine what is known of the hazard so that protective equipment may be used.

- *What will be the effect on the responders and on the incident if the hazard is not mitigated?* Responders may be killed or injured. This will impact the EMS system as well as the surviving responders on the scene.
- *What protection will be needed to help with this hazard?* Responders may need special suits or equipment. If this is the case, crews will need additional training prior to the response. EMS agencies must ensure that their responders have the required equipment and training to deal with the hazard.

- *What about sheltering-in-place?* Sheltering-in-place may require an increase in staffing or it may require transport units to stay on scene longer. This will have a serious effect on the overall EMS system. During preplanning, organizations may need to ensure mutual aid or recall staff.
- *Will sheltering-in-place put the residents/patients in a potentially hazardous condition?* During sheltering-in-place, it may become necessary to move residents/patients with little time available. To address this issue, EMS should ensure mutual aid or recall staff.
- *Is there anything needed to protect people, both the public and the responders?* EMS must assess the need for specialized equipment and training.
- *Will weather either positively or negatively affect the hazard?* Cold temperatures will drive vapor clouds downward, while warmer temperatures will cause vapor to rise upward in a plume. Excessive heat or cold as well as wetness from rain can also intensify the impact of certain hazards. EMS preplans should provide for tents, other facilities or capabilities to treat people, or a plan to move people if the weather makes a hazard "mobile."
- *Will rain or increased heat or cold weather make the hazard more or less safe?* Again, EMS agencies should ensure proper specialized equipment and training, while assessing the need to evacuate more people, depending on the agent and its characteristics.
- *What routes for access and egress are available?* A particular hazard might block additional incoming units or transportation to a receiving hospital. EMS should consider incorporating prepared secondary routes for access and egress, to facilitate any necessary movement.
- *What else does EMS need to know?* Through coordination with other agencies, more information will become available and any additional information will be identified.

Basically, the question is: What assistance is needed, by whom, to accomplish what tasks?

## Capability Analysis

Once EMS has compiled a list of the hazards, they must ask the following: What capability is available to mitigate or deal with these hazards? What are the specific risks, potential benefits, and costs of a hazard?

Just because there is a hazard does not mean that there is a requirement to spend thousands or millions of dollars to deal with it. EMS must address the following: Is mitigation of a specific hazard or combination of hazards beyond local capabilities? Other questions related to local capabilities must be answered as well.

- Is there training available to overcome a hazard or combination of hazards, either locally, regionally, or nationally?
- What equipment or technology is needed to overcome or mitigate the hazards identified?
- If new equipment or technology is needed, can it be acquired locally? If not, can it be acquired through rental, regional asset sharing, or mutual aid? If the capability is not local, is it somewhere close by? Has the capable, nearby agency been coordinated with? If not, what needs to be done in order to acquire the necessary capability?
- What can be done and how long will it take to mitigate the hazard? Depending on the hazard, will local capabilities be available to contain and deal with the hazard until help arrives in 2 hours, 3 hours, or 2 days?

EMS agencies must also ask whether there is redundancy in the capability. Some business models look at redundancy as a waste of effort and money. Experience has shown, however, that redundancy in an emergency operation is beneficial. It is a common practice in fireground operations, and it is a useful tool for EMS in large or complex incidents.

With all that has been mentioned, it is easy for EMS agencies to become stunned at the amount of information needed to effectively preplan. This should not halt the EMS preplanning process. A tenet of planning is that a good and actionable plan developed now beats a perfect plan developed later. If a good plan exists that meets 85% or 90% of an EMS agency's current response needs, responders can move forward with training and coordination. The rest of the plan can be updated later as information is developed and worked out.

## Selected References

Auf Der Heide, E: *Disaster Response: Principles of Preparation and Coordination*. St. Louis, MO: Mosby-Year Book, Inc.; 1989.

Baker, D: Civilian exposure to toxic agents: Emergency medical response. *Prehosp Disaster Med* 2004;19(2):174–178.

Centers for Disease Control and Prevention: *The Public Health Response to Biological and Chemical Terrorism*. US Department of Health and Human Services; 2001.

Cuny, F: Cuny memorial continuing education series, principles of disaster management: Lesson 1. *Prehosp Disaster Med* 1998;13(1):88–92.

Cuny, F: Cuny memorial continuing education series, principles of disaster management: Lesson 2. *Prehosp Disaster Med* 1998;13(2–4):63–79.

Deitchman, S: What have we learned? Needs assessment. *Prehosp Disaster Med* 2005;20(6):468–470.

Doyle, CJ: Mass casualty incident. Integration with prehospital care. *Emergency Medicine Clinics of North America* 1990;8(1):163–175.

Drabek, T and Hoetmer, G: *Emergency Management: Principles and Practice for Local Government*. Washington, D.C.: International City/County Management Association; 1996.

*Federal Response to Hurricane Katrina: Lessons learned*. Washington, D.C.: The White House; February 23, 2006.

FEMA: *Guide for All Hazards Planning Emergency Operations Planning*. Washington D.C.: FEMA; September, 1996.

FEMA: *Assistance to Firefighters Grant Program*. http://www.firegrantsupport.com. Accessed January 15, 2009.

Hooke, W and Rodgers, P, eds.: *Public Health Risks of Disasters: Communication, Infrastructure and Preparedness*. Washington, D.C.: The National Academies Press; 2005.

International Association of Fire Fighters and International Association of Fire Chiefs: *Everyone Comes Home Initiative*. http://www.everyonegoeshome.com. Accessed January 16, 2009.

Joint Commission on Accreditation of Healthcare Organizations: *Standing Together: An Emergency Planning Guide for America's Communities*. Washington, D.C.: JCAHO; 2005.

Kerins, D and Cortacans, HP: *Pre-Planning and Preparedness Pay Off; New Jersey EMS Response to US Airways Hudson River Crash*. http://www.JEMS.com. Accessed February 2, 2009.

Lintu, N, Health, M, et al.: Reactions to cold exposure emphasize the need for weather protection in prehospital care: An experimental study. *Prehosp Disaster Med* 2006;21(5):316–320.

Maguire, B, Dean, S, et al.: Epidemic and bioterrorism preparation among emergency medical services systems. *Prehosp Disaster Med* 2007;22(3):237–242.

Manning, F and Goldfrank, L, ed.: *Preparing for Terrorism: Tools for Evaluating the Metropolitan Medical Response System Program*. Committee on Evaluation of the Metropolitan Medical Response System, Board on Health Sciences Policy. Washington, D.C.: The National Academies Press; 2002.

Moles, TM: Emergency medical services systems and HAZMAT major incidents. *Resuscitation* 1999;42(2):103–116.

Rowitz, L: *Public Health for the 21st Century: The Prepared Leader*. Sudbury, MA: Jones and Bartlett Publishers; 2006.

United States Department of Homeland Security: *Department of Homeland Security Spending Documents 2007*. http://www.dhs.gov. Accessed December 30, 2008.

United States Fire Administration. *FA-166 Risk Management Practices in the Fire Service.* Emmitsburg, MD: USFA; December, 1996.

United States National Committee for the Decade for Natural Disaster Reduction: *A Safer Future: Reducing the Impacts of Natural Disasters.* National Research Council; 1991.

Vilke, G, Smith, A, et al.: Impact of the San Diego county firestorm on emergency medical services. *Prehosp Disaster Med* 2006;21(5):353–358.

Waldman, R: What have we learned? Filling gaps in available services. *Prehosp Disaster Med* 2005;20(6):475–479.

World Health Organization: *Studies on ED Planning and Hazards.* http://www.who.int. Accessed February 2, 2009.

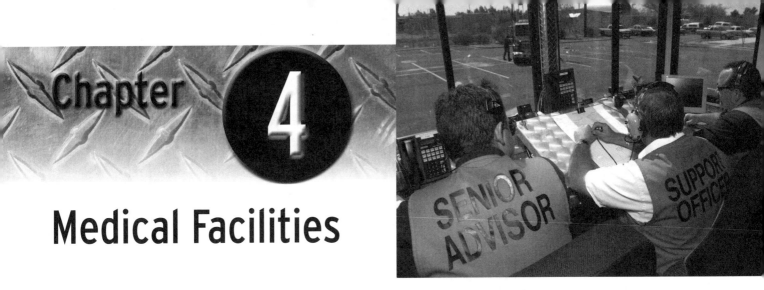

# Chapter 4

# Medical Facilities

## EMS Preplanning for Medical Facilities

In terms of planning, medical facilities are of special concern to emergency medical services (EMS) agencies because they present numerous hazards, and the conditions of people residing within vary greatly. Patients may have unique disabilities, be acutely ill, or be in an intensive care setting. Additionally, medical facilities will have large populations of patients with mobility concerns. Patients may be ambulatory, be of disabled or impaired mobility, have communication difficulties, or suffer from chronic conditions that restrict their movement. Certain patients may also be technology-dependent, such as those connected to ventilators.

When gathering preplanning data on medical facilities, the major points of consideration will be the day-to-day operations of the facility (business functions) and the medical environment (patient care and treatment functions). Medical facilities pose a preplanning concern to EMS because they are community assets, and the EMS system is dependent on having an operational facility where EMS providers can transfer the care of prehospital patients. The effectiveness of an EMS system also is contingent upon the ability to mobilize patients and resources between facilities, should the need arise in cases such as a disaster. Even a temporary loss of function for a medical facility has a significant impact on the entire local EMS system.

Consider the following example: If a tornado strikes the only hospital in an EMS provider's jurisdiction that is capable of providing cardiac catheterization procedures to acutely ill heart attack victims, the patient's survivability may be affected by a longer transport time to a facility that is further away and unscathed by tornado or storm activity. The hospital struck by the tornado may also need to be evacuated, which would necessitate an EMS response to assist with moving patients to another facility or providing care at an alternate site capable of temporarily accommodating patients. Alternate locations may include an indoor stadium or convention hall receiving facilities. Although it is impossible to be very specific on what should be in place with the alternate locations due to variables of number of patients, conditions, medical equipment needs, and so forth, key features of the alternate temporary locations would include access and egress for ambulances, equipment storage space, a treatment section, an administrative section, and protection from weather extremes. It is important to protect patients from the weather, as many of these patients may be compromised and unable to regulate internal body temperature. Other environmental issues to consider are direct sunlight, wind, rain, and noise.

According to the Joint Commission on Accreditation of Healthcare Organizations (JCAHO), there are three aspects that define medical facility emergencies. One, two, or all three of these may be encountered at any given incident involving a medical facility. The first type of emergency is one that disrupts the environment of care. For example, an emergency incident could cause damages to the organization's buildings and grounds. This could be due to a natural or manmade disaster.

A second type of emergency disrupts care and treatment through a loss of utilities. For most EMS agencies and responders, the frame of reference with regard to disasters or incidents centers on a catastrophic event, such as a fire or explosion. Imagine, however, how a loss of water might affect a medical facility's ability to function. In a facility without running water, there are no operational toilets. This condition poses a threat to general hygiene by disrupting hand washing for operating room procedures and preventing the regular cleaning of facilities. Loss of water, furthermore, often couples with a loss of power. Facilities experiencing these difficulties must rely upon the use of backup means, such as generators.

The third element in the definition describes a medical facility emergency as something that causes an increase in demand for organizational service. A significant influx of patients could be considered a disaster if the organization is unable to deal with the large increase in patient care needs. This type of increase was seen with the 1995 Tokyo Sarin attacks as well as the 2005 bombings in London.

Being aware of the hospital's view of what constitutes an emergency can help EMS to understand the various functions that medical facilities must maintain for the provision of emergency care. Three key components affect the hospital's ability to maintain continuity of operations: census, capacity, and capability.

The census is the current count or tally of patients admitted to the hospital (see **Figure 4-1**). Some facilities weigh this number against the average number of patients per day, month, or year. This assists in tracking from year to year if a facility's admission rates are up or down in comparison to prior data. Census is also the mechanism by which hospitals plan for "seasonal" illnesses and admission rates for outbreaks such as influenza. For example, a hospital may have data that reflects a higher admission rate or census during the winter months for respiratory illnesses. In response to this data, they increase staffing needs to accommodate the census change. Almost all facilities have to record and report this data to state agencies. They may report that they have an average of 500 beds per month that are being used.

A facility's capacity is based upon the beds available for admission in each separate area of the hospital with staffing currently available to care for the patients admitted (see **Figure 4-2**). The obstetrics wing of the hospital, for instance, may have the current capacity to admit and staff beds for five patient admissions.

---

## Skilled Nursing/Assisted Living Facility Census Tracking Form

The information provided on this form is voluntary and will be used by the Anytown Fire Department for planning purposes only. The Anytown Fire Department acknowledges the cooperation of the facility named herein and extends its appreciation to the facility in assisting the Anytown Fire Department in the protection of all of the citizens in the city.

Date: _____

### Facility Information
Facility Name: _____
Facility Type:
  ☐  Skilled Nursing Facility     ☐  Assisted Living Facility
  ☐  Independent Living
Address:_____, Anytown, TX, _____
Contact Information: _____ Telephone #: (____) ____-_____

### Census Information
Total Census: _____ Facility Available Beds: _____
Total Bed-Bound Persons: _____
Number of Bariatric Persons: _____ (> 350 lbs)
Total Number of Dementia/Secured Persons: _____ (Need one-on-one care if moved)
Number of persons needing ventilation support (eg, ventilators): _____

### Additional Comments
_____
_____
_____
_____

Thank you for your cooperation.
Please call AFD EMS at (XXX) XXX-XXXX with any questions.
Please fax to Anytown Fire Department EMS Division at (XXX) XXX-XXXX.

**Figure 4-1** Sample census tracking form.

The hospital's capacity waxes and wanes as its census increases or decreases and as patients are released from rooms or upgraded to a higher level of patient care (eg, being transferred from a medical "floor" bed to an intensive care unit). The capacity is also dependent upon the number of patients treated in the emergency department and how many are admitted to the hospital rather than released to their residence.

Capability refers to a medical facility's ability to potentially contain a greater number of patients than it holds during day-to-day operations. For example, the obstetrics wing of the hospital might have a total of 10 rooms, and each can potentially contain two patient beds. Therefore, the obstetrics wing is capable of admitting 20 patients. Because each hospital has a certain numbers of beds, it is capable of admitting only a certain number of patients. It must also be taken into

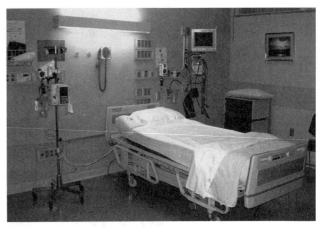

**Figure 4-2** Capacity refers to the quantity of patients a medical facility may accommodate, based on the number of available beds and staffing abilities.

consideration that a hospital's capability may be an exception to its "normal" daily operations, as private rooms may become double occupancy. During emergency conditions, hospitals may be able to provide additional space not designated as patient care areas for taking in additional patients. Examples of such spaces include lobbies, auditoriums, and classrooms.

The total capacity of a medical facility is based on the capability of space for patient admissions and on the staffing ability. A wing or unit may not have the staff support to fully admit to its total capability. This is directly correlated to the current health care worker shortage experience nationwide. As a result of this shortage, in the United States, most EMS systems with a local hospital emergency room or emergency department are running near capacity most of the time. A large surge of people would disrupt the ability of the hospital or any medical facility to deal with and treat those people. Because medical facilities are running at near capacity, or experience decreased capability when they shut wings down, this is of concern to EMS. A medical facility may have a total capacity of 1,000 beds, but due to economic reasons they may only have 500 beds available and staff to care for 500 patients. A facility that may be a 1,000-bed facility will not necessarily have 1,000 beds available for use. Regular monitoring of local medical facility capacity by the EMS system is advisable and will be helpful during normal and mass-casualty incidents (MCIs). Agencies that incorporate this into their preplan will be better equipped to respond when an incident occurs that affects a medical facility's ability to provide care.

## Internal Disaster Plans for Medical Facilities

Emergency program managers employed by hospitals create their medical facility preplans in a similar fashion as those models previously mentioned in Chapter 2. A hospital's "All-Hazards Emergency Operations Plan" outlines the hospital's strategy for response and recovery. The emergency operations plan (EOP) provides overall direction and coordination of the response structure. It indicates the processes and procedures to be used, while guiding implementation of the incident command system (ICS), communication, and coordination. Critical EOP elements to be considered by EMS agencies when interfacing with hospital planners include management and planning; departmental and/or organizational roles and responsibilities before, during, and after emergencies; health and medical operations; internal and external communication; logistics; finance; equipment; and patient tracking. EMS preplanning for response to a hospital emergency should focus on evacuation, triage, transport, and assisting the hospital to maintain and/or regain its continuity of operations.

All medical facilities, regardless of size or location, are required to have internal disaster plans. According to state regulations, a hospital's accreditation is contingent upon having the appropriate plans and personnel in place to execute the plans. A plan not only needs to be constructed, but it also needs to be trained and exercised. It must also be revised accordingly as gaps between standard procedure and current response needs are identified. EMS agencies must investigate what gaps are known by the facility and should also look into any mutual aid agreements established to mitigate the gaps. It is also important for EMS agencies to know when a facility's plan was created and how recently it was updated.

EMS responders must always be aware that medical facilities may be the site of an incident or an emergency, or they may be the receiving facility of patients from an incident or another facility. The hospital's ability to maintain its continuity of operations is dependent upon its capabilities prior to, during, and recovering from an incident.

Hospitals have static roles in emergencies or disasters. According to FEMA's guide on "Nine Hazard All-Emergency Operation Plans," hospitals are mandated to carry out their intended disaster plan based on their capabilities. It is the responsibility of the EMS agency to determine what the capabilities of a certain facility are. In the preplanning phase, EMS must develop assumptions about a facility, while documenting the source and basis of these assumptions.

## Roles and Responsibilities Before, During, and After a Medical Facility Emergency

In combination with the hospital's internal disaster plan and identified capabilities or gaps, a facility should also outline and predetermine the roles and responsibilities of its personnel. This is normally accomplished using an organizational chart with descriptions of duties for each position. Most facilities also designate roles and responsibilities that will be delegated to outside persons or agencies, such as the local EMS provider transferring patients to another facility if a full evacuation is initiated. EMS agencies also need to be cognizant that their normal roles and responsibilities (to the 9-1-1 system or other contracts) continue despite a disaster response. There will be a significant demand in the use of EMS resources once an evacuation occurs.

EMS agencies must formulate a preplan, outlining the actions to be taken to initiate and support a shift from the hospital to the field or vice versa. It is important for agencies to foresee the effect such a shift will have on their staffing and resources. For instance, if EMS is staffing to assist a facility at one level, and the facility's needs increase because of evacuation, the agency must have a plan allowing them to meet those needs without drastically disrupting normal EMS operations.

## Medical Facility Emergency Operations

Hospitals are charged with the task of coordinating with other area hospitals to allow both facilities to receive and transfer patients, in an effort for both facilities to maintain some continuity of care. Hospitals are also obligated to establish and maintain communication between the field and other medical communities or facilities. This duty mandates that the facility be incorporated into other local and regional response plans, in the event of a large incident where they will have to work in coordination with other agencies and medical facilities. EMS agencies must determine what hospitals located in their jurisdiction are able to assist each other at the onset of and throughout a disaster. It is also important for EMS to assess what capabilities these facilities have to move their operations to a field setting.

A crucial component in maintaining operations is a facility's ability to funnel timely and appropriate information through the proper channels. Information regarding a facility's current situation and its ability or inability to continue "business as usual" needs to be provided to the public information officer (PIO). The PIO is charged with providing information to the public and to patients about what is happening, what the facility is capable of, or whether it is incapable of handling a certain incident. The PIO should let the public and responders know when not to request the facility's services and also suggest to them where else they may seek treatment when the facility's operations have been disturbed.

EMS is responsible for securing contact information for the PIOs for medical facilities in an agency's jurisdiction. Before incorporating a facility into an EMS preplan, an agency must first determine what other response agencies depend upon the facility in question. Furthermore, EMS must always communicate to medical facilities regarding their involvement in EMS preplans.

### Internal and External Communication

Embedded within a medical facility's disaster plan, it is critical for EMS responders to understand the established communications plan. Responders must know how the medical facility works in terms of communication during a disaster, and they must identify a primary and alternate method of communication. Inside the communication plan, a facility identifies both its internal and external modes of communication. Internal communication may be conducted by telephone, pager, or radio. When testing the overall EOP of a facility, response agencies need to test their interoperable communications during training and exercises. A medical facility's communications plan should indicate when alternate modes of communication are needed. The need for this shift may depend on incident type, patient type, patient volume, or time of day.

Communications have been shown in almost every incident after action report (AAR), planning session review, and training session review to be a critical component that most often breaks down and causes further failures within an incident. With proper training, this vulnerability can be prepared for and mitigated, from a response perspective. It is critical, when a medical facility expects responders to operate within a medical facility, that EMS understands the facility's communication capabilities. Agencies should preplan on the assumption that one mode will fail, and develop a secondary and possibly tertiary mode of communication. EMS should also be aware of the conditions under which an alternate means of communication will need to be used during a medical facility disaster response. Protocol must be in place to ensure that everyone working within the communication network is promptly notified of the shift to the alternate method.

## Logistics Planning for Medical Facilities

In planning and in real-time responsibility during an incident, the role of logistics is to coordinate the right people with the right resources. The level of EMS support needed to respond to a medical facility during an incident depends on the number and type of patients who need to be cared for or transferred to another facility. It also depends on the resources currently available at the facility.

EMS agencies must remain cognizant of their roles and responsibilities to the communities they serve; during the planning stages with a medical facility, agencies should not obligate resources that will diminish their ability to meet their contractual agreements. The ability of the medical facility and EMS responses to sustain their efforts should be mapped out in the plan. For example: The disaster plan of a medical facility for an evacuation needing the assistance from an EMS agency may outline that the resources from the responders will be needed for up to 72 hours. It may also include further details on the number of people and resources the agency will need to bring to the facility.

## Assessing the Need for EMS Resources

When planning from a logistics perspective, medical facilities need to consider time of day and normal business hours in relation to the number of people in the facility. As one would expect, normal business hours are from 8:00 am to 5:00 pm, Monday through Friday. Medical facilities tend to have more people in the facility during this time frame because of the administrative staff, housekeeping, food services, and all the other ancillary people of the facility. When creating a disaster plan, the ratio of staff to patients and total facility staff needs to be assessed. EMS should ask the following questions about staffing when preplanning for a medical facility:

- How many staff members are available per shift?
- Is there a "call in/call back" procedure in place for requesting off-duty personnel to return to the facility?
- Are there any agreements for surge, such as contracts to have supplemental staff come in case of emergency? For instance, is home health, public health, or anyone else available to supplement their staffing?

EMS agencies must assess the logistics of medical facilities in their jurisdiction to determine which facilities will potentially request EMS equipment. It is important for agencies to preplan what type of equipment will be requested by each facility, how long it will be in use, and how much of the EMS equipment will need to be contributed. Next, protocol must be developed for distributing EMS supplies to the facility in need. Agencies may look into securing a surge pack from their medical supply vendor based on the facility's anticipated needs.

## Special Population Patient Needs

Another planning point of consideration is patient types. In medical care facilities, the number of patients served and the types of patients regularly admitted to the facility need to be reflected in the plan. This is especially true with regard to evacuation. A facility's patient population will include both ambulatory patients (who can move by themselves or with minimal assistance) and nonambulatory patients (who require assistance) (see **Figure 4-3**). Pediatric patients also require additional assistance in movement and supervision. This is in addition to their need for specialized care equipment.

Special population patient types also include critical care patients or high-acuity patients. Based on the number of high-acuity patients, EMS agencies can postulate how long the facility will be able to sustain operations during an internal disaster. If a facility has bariatric patients, these individuals may require the resources of numerous staff members to move them efficiently. Bariatric patients may also occupy specialty beds, some of which weigh in excess of 800 or 900 pounds. This is in addition to the weight of the patient and may create a situation in which responders must transport up to two tons. Ventilator-dependent patients will require the use of an electrical circuit to maintain their equipment needs. In preparation for loss of electrical power at a medical facility, a preplan should indicate battery supply or tasking of 1:1 patient care to medical personnel, to provide manual ventilation support to the patients. During preplanning, EMS agencies must take into consideration how long providers will be able to provide ventilation support.

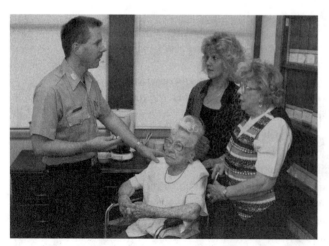

**Figure 4-3** In preplanning for a medical facility, EMS agencies must take into consideration its population of nonambulatory patients who will require assistance during an evacuation.

## Case Study

### Background

In August 2005 Hurricane Katrina forced the evacuation of thousands of people from their homes in the Gulf Coast region of the United States. One group of people especially impacted by the storm was nursing home residents in western Louisiana and eastern Texas. Hundreds if not thousands of nursing home residents were moved inland to receiving nursing homes without prior planning, mostly due to a lack of experience in large-scale evacuations. Residents were loaded onto buses or other means of transportation, and were moved toward the inland areas of Texas. In many cases, they headed for the Dallas/Fort Worth metroplex.

One of the suburban cities around Dallas was selected to receive the evacuated residents. This city has a robust EMS system, a large professional fire department (EMS falls under the fire department), and a population of approximately 230,000. One of the nursing homes was selected to receive incoming residents, mostly because its location only a few blocks from an interstate highway afforded excellent access for the buses bringing the residents into town.

The nursing home selected is a unique facility as it has three wings of ventilator patients, totaling approximately 50, as well as an Alzheimer's wing with a resident population of 25 residents. The total population for the facility was approximately 175 residents including those already mentioned.

### The Preplan

Several battalion chiefs or shift officers were asked about the preplan for the facility and when pressed could offer a single-page fire preplan. The preplan consisted of projected locations for the first-, second-, and third-arriving engines (pumpers), the first and second ladder trucks, the EMS supervisor, the battalion chief, and one ambulance that would be dedicated to either fire suppression activities or incident rehabilitation duties once there was evidence of no patients. This is a normal assignment for the department.

The building sat on a major road through the city with three to four traffic lanes on each side depending how far away from a corner for right hand turns.

The plan did not consider where residents could be temporarily placed, who would ventilate the approximately 50 ventilator-dependent residents or how to handle 25 Alzheimer's or other mentally impaired residents, let alone how to move that many residents out in any coordinated fashion.

The facility itself had a contract with a private (non-municipal) EMS agency who had a fleet of six ambulances available at peak operating hours.

### The Results

No deaths or negative outcomes from the facility because the facility did not have to evacuate.

Several procedures and policies were put in place to correct the plan and the response. One of the significant outcomes was a citywide forum between the fire department, EMS, and the eight nursing homes in the city. The forum came up with one form which could address the needs of EMS and the facility so that all could utilize one form. Additionally, the fire department developed a census form that the nursing homes voluntarily completed every month, which told the fire department critical planning information such as how many ventilator or other technology-dependent residents were in the facility, the number of residents over 350 lbs or bariatric residents, and how many Alzheimer's or mentally challenged residents were in the facility. A mini–mental-evaluation (MME) form was also developed, guiding responders through a quick assessment of individual residents' mental status (see **Figure 4-4**). This information was also shared with the city emergency management agency so the agency had a realistic number of how many nursing home residents were in the city so that appropriate resources could be requested based on numbers of people, not number of facilities.

---

### Mini-Mental-Evaluation (MME) Form

**Orientation**
| | | |
|---|---|---|
| 5 | ( ) | Ask: "What is the (year, season, date, day, or month)?" |
| 5 | ( ) | Ask: "What (state, country, town, hospital, or floor) are we located in?" |

**Registration**
| | | |
|---|---|---|
| 3 | ( ) | Name 3 objects. Then ask the patient to recite all 3 after you have said them. Give patient 1 second to say each. Give 1 point for each correct answer. Repeat the items until he or she learns all 3. Count the number of trials and record. Trials: _____ |

**Attention and Calculation**
| | | |
|---|---|---|
| 5 | ( ) | Serial 7s: 1 point for each correct answer. Stop after 5 answers. Alternatively, ask the patient to spell "world" backwards. |

**Recall**
| | | |
|---|---|---|
| 3 | ( ) | Ask for the 3 objects repeated above. Give 1 point for each correct answer. |

**Language**
| | | |
|---|---|---|
| 2 | ( ) | Ask the patient to name a pencil and watch. |
| 1 | ( ) | Have the patient repeat the following: "No ifs, ands, or buts." |
| 3 | ( ) | Ask the patient to follow a 3-stage command: "Take a paper in your hand, fold it in half, and put it on the floor." |
| 1 | ( ) | Ask the patient to read and obey the following: **CLOSE YOUR EYES** |
| 1 | ( ) | Ask the patient to write a sentence. |
| 1 | ( ) | Copy the design shown: |

**Total:** _____
The higher the score, the more intact the mental capabilities
(30 = Highest Score).

**Assess the patient's level of consciousness along a continuum:**
☐ Alert   ☐ Drowsy   ☐ Stupor   ☐ Coma

**Figure 4-4** Sample MME form.

## Tracking the Distribution of EMS Resources

During initiation of a facility's disaster plan, maintenance of record keeping and diligent tracking of expenditures are imperative. Oftentimes, the role of finance/administration is completing necessary paperwork and documentation to obtain reimbursement after the response phase of a disaster ends and the recovery phase begins. EMS agencies included in a medical facility's disaster plan need to be made aware in advance of their roles in record keeping for financial responsibilities.

After being informed of their involvement in the finance aspect of emergency response, an agency should establish a system for tracking EMS resource use and expenditure to be incorporated into its preplans for the medical facility. An agency may wish to document travel time to and from the facility, including mileage, to be reimbursed for transporting supplies. Responders charged with the task of bringing resources to the facility in need should clock in and out during the response, with whoever is responsible for maintaining those logs or records.

EMS agencies also need to be made aware in advance of any items that a medical facility may plan to use from its existing supply. Additionally, agencies should consider stocking a cache of supplies in advance for use during disasters, while instituting a plan to rotate items with limited shelf life or an expiration date. During an agency's initial assessment of a facility, it should be determined whether space is available to cache EMS supplies in advance of an incident. Examples of items to be cached include oxygen bottles, batteries, electrodes for cardiac monitors, intravenous (IV) maintenance supplies, IV fluids, self-care kits, bandaging and splinting supplies, food, and water. It is difficult to extrapolate how many supplies may be needed for a potential disaster response. A good starting point for determining this, however, is to plot an agency's regular usage. This provides a baseline of yearly, monthly, and weekly rates for usage of various items.

During preplanning, EMS must consider how they will resupply what will be used by a medical facility during a disaster. Will it be accomplished organically—through the agency's normal restock process—or through another, emergency restock process? Will the medical facility facilitate restocking, for instance, by having IV bags, IV start kits, and/or electrodes available?

# Incorporating Patient Tracking into an EMS Preplan

When it has been determined that a medical facility will be unable to maintain continuity of operations during a particular disaster—warranting the distribution of patients to other facilities—it is imperative for EMS to consider the mechanism of how patients will be treated and tracked. During preplanning, EMS agencies must ask the following questions regarding the tracking of patients: Will triage tags be utilized to prioritize patient care (see **Figure 4-5**)? Will any available medical charts and documentation on patients travel with them throughout the incident (see **Figure 4-6**)? Are there alternative documents that are utilized during activation of the disaster plan? Great efforts should be made in planning for the transportation of the right patients to the right facilities while maintaining continuity of care.

Consider the following example: A patient needs to be moved from a level one trauma facility to another level one trauma center, rather than to a local community hospital. The local community hospital may not have resources to deal with such a high-acuity patient. Also to be taken into consideration is how to reunite families separated during an incident. EMS agencies should determine, during preplanning, what information will be made available to these families. Preplanning the strategies the facility and EMS will employ to track and distribute patients is imperative to the success of the response and evacuation.

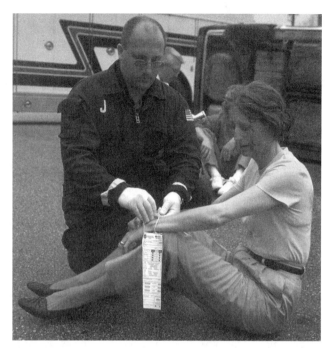

**Figure 4-5** Triage is the sorting of two or more patients based on the severity of their conditions to establish priorities for care based on available resources.

## Fatality Management

Any disaster has the potential to cause loss of life. Health care providers' quest is to provide life safety and life-saving efforts. Despite providers' best attempts, people may die. Medical facility disaster plans need to include contingencies for those who die during the incident. EMS agencies must consider where the deceased will be taken, how they will be identified, who will process the remains, and whether or not family members will be permitted to view the remains.

## Decontamination

Part of the coordinated response effort needs to be focused on how patients will be decontaminated during an incident. One point to address is whether the decontamination area is mobile or fixated and whether additional resources from local responders will need to be utilized. Every medical facility has hazardous materials stored within the confines of its building. EMS agencies must determine where normal hazardous material storage is in relation to patient rooms. Is there a potential for a hazardous material leak? If decontamination is needed during a response, how will it be accomplished? Will hospital staff, EMS personnel, or hazardous materials personnel be responsible for decontamination?

## Safety and Security

The role of a medical facility's safety and security personnel during disaster is to ensure that the perimeter and access to the facility is maintained. In instances where a facility must shut down the incoming flow of additional patients, it is difficult to maintain vigilance. The security

## Universal Emergent In-Patient Transfer Form

Date: _____    Room/Bed: _____

Patient Name: _____, _____ _____
            Last        First        MI

DOB: ___/___/____    SSN: ___-___-____
    mm/dd/yyyy

Family Contact: _____ Telephone #: (___) ___-_____

Contacted: □ Yes   □ No

Treating Physician: _____ Telephone #: (___) ____-_____

Facility Transferring Patient: _____ Telephone #: (___) ____-_____

Transferring to: _____    Reason: □ Hosp.   □ ED   □ Evacuation

Patient DNR: □ Yes   □ No    Original DNR on file at originating facility? □ Yes   □ No

Patient ID Band on Patient: □ Yes   □ No    # _____

Bariatric? □ Yes   □ No    Ventilator-Dependent? □ Yes   □ No

Primary Condition(s): □ Cardiac    □ Diabetic    □ Respiratory/COPD

                    □ Seizures    □ Alzheimer's

                    Other: _____

MME Score: _____    Normal Mental Status: □ Alert   □ Confused

Patient Needs One-on-One Care: □ Yes   □ No    If yes, explain: _____

Allergies: _____ NKDA

Activity Level: □ Walk without assistance    □ Walk with assistance (cane, crutches)

                □ Geriatric chair/Wheelchair   □ Bed-bound

---

**Please complete the bottom half in writing, using either blue or black ink.**

MAR Attached: □ Yes   □ No    Primary Medication(s)*: _____

Last Vital Signs (VS): _____    Time Taken: _____

    Last Prior VS: _____    Time Taken: _____

    Last Medications Given: _____    Time Taken: _____

Oxygen Required: □ Yes   □ No    Lpm: ___    Via: □ NC   □ NRB   □ ET   □ Other

    Special Equipment Needed: □ Yes   □ No    If yes, list: _____

    Other information: _____

Person Requesting Transfer: _____    □ DR   □ Nurse   □ Admin.

                            □ FD   □ Other

*Not needed if MAR attached

**Figure 4-6** Sample patient tracking form.

personnel are also crucial for establishing and maintaining control over the traffic flow into and out of the grounds of a facility. Both pedestrian and vehicular traffic flow need to be considered. Plans should encompass access and egress with alternate routes and also include the need for decontamination.

During preplanning, EMS agencies must ask the following questions pertaining to facility safety and security: How many floors does the facility have? Where are the security checkpoints? Where are all routes of entry and exit? Where are ramps and parking areas located? What areas of the facility are regularly secured or unsecured? What modes of transportation will be utilized to provide emergency care and to transport patients away from the incident scene? Will buses and aircraft be needed or utilized?

Some facilities will require an expansion of security personnel's role during an activation of a disaster plan. In addition to their regular duties, they may be asked to assist with minimal patient care duties. Providing the appropriate medical training to these personnel prior to the activation of the plan is essential.

## Coordination With External Agencies

As previously mentioned, the process of planning is

all about building relationships between response partners and predetermining the roles and responsibilities of each agency. Medical facilities that are realistic in their planning and that are acutely aware of any deficiencies they have will be the most successful in reaching out to their community response partners in order to provide the greatest life safety measures. Most agencies are willing to buy into the plan and offer their assistance when disaster occurs; predetermining responders' roles and including them in the planning will serve to augment the control of a chaotic situation.

Key issues for EMS to consider: What is the agency's role in a medical facility's disaster plan? Will EMS responders be asked to conduct duties outside their normal span of control? Is there a plan to deal with the worst case scenario? How will EMS interface with other response partners? Who will establish and/or maintain incident/area command?

A facility's successful EOP should be consistent with local, state, and regional EOPs, adhere to the fundamental tenets found in the National Response Plan (NRP), and include hazard- or incident-specific guidance documents. These articulate how the EOP is applied to a particular hazard or incident. The hazards of significance to the hospital are identified through the hazard vulnerability analysis (HVA).

## Hazard Vulnerability Analysis

The HVA is a key element of the EOP. It drives threat- and incident-specific planning by identifying, prioritizing, and defining threats that may impact business operations. The HVA provides specific steps to reduce the impact of threat occurrence and ensures the ongoing business functions of the medical facility.

The hazard analysis assesses probability and impact. Probability is the likelihood of an event occurrence. It is calculated by retrospective assessment of event frequency. This calculation can be predicted by estimation of risk factors. Impact is the severity or damage caused by a threat and the effect on human lives, business operations, infrastructure, and environmental conditions. The hazard analysis also includes risk. Risk is the calculated score of the interactions between probability and impact for each threat. Risk can be reduced by threat-mitigation activities.

A hospital's HVA should be developed in conjunction with community responders. By fostering this relationship between the medical facility and local responders, the combined efforts serve to improve preparedness and response activities, enhance multidisciplinary and agency coordination, and maximize use and effectiveness of limited resources.

### Hospital Emergency Incident Command System

The Hospital Emergency Incident Command System (HEICS) is an emergency management system that employs a logical management structure, defined responsibilities, clear reporting channels, and a common nomenclature to help unify hospitals with other emergency responders. HEICS is very similar in structure to the ICS widely utilized by the public safety community—the only differences are that the positions delegated within the organizational structure are specific to maintaining the continuity of operations for a medical facility. EMS providers

> **Preplanning Practices**
>
> Certain preplanning considerations specifically relate to hospitals and nursing homes. Several studies and a few literature reviews found that there were 275 evacuations from 1971 to 1999. With an average of 21, 33 were recorded in 1994, the year of the Northridge, CA earthquake. Of all the evacuations, 23 were attributed to static fire, followed by 18% attributed to hazardous materials threats, 14% to hurricanes, 13% to human threats, 16% to external fires, 6% to floods, and 5% to utility failure. Clearly, more than 50% of hospital evacuations occurred because of hazards outside of the hospital or from human intruders. Hospitals are susceptible to many hazards, and EMS agencies should be aware of them.

should be familiar with the organizational structure of a hospital's plan, because they will need to be aware of who is in the incident command position and who may be directing their response upon arrival at a medical facility. Additionally, those who are trained to HEICS standards are taught to create incident planning guides (IPGs). The IPGs assist hospitals to plan for potential disaster-related incidents, evaluate existing EOPs, and develop needed plans and procedures.

IPGs include planning considerations for operational periods and response phases defined as follows:

- Immediate: 0 to 2 hours
- Intermediate: 2 to 12 hours
- Extended: More than 12 hours
- Demobilization/system recovery

The operational periods and response phases included in an IPG are significant to EMS providers, as the agency's response plan will need to be in alignment with the hospital's plan or expectation. For example: If a hospital states in its IPG that a response to an internal flood will warrant the need for an intermediate response, EMS providers may be asked to provide services and support to the hospital for up to 12 hours.

In an effort to augment a hospital's ability to test its capabilities and preparedness activities related to the plans, HEICS provides scenario-based IPGs, including 14 external scenarios based on the national planning scenarios and 13 internal hospital scenarios. These scenarios provide a foundation for training and exercising with jurisdictional partners to test the plans prior to a time of activation. EMS providers should remain engaged with not only their supervising hospital but with all hospitals in their jurisdiction so that the providers are familiar with the hospital's intended role for the agency in an emergency response to their medical facility. EMS providers can benefit from being involved in the hospital's training exercise, because this gives the agency an opportunity to evaluate its plans.

## Medical Facility Hazards Requiring Evacuation

Several types of hazards pose a threat to medical facilities, which require evacuation of patients and staff. These can be divided between internal and external emergencies and disasters.

### Internal Emergencies and Disasters

Fire, smoke, hazardous materials release, or irritant fumes in the following areas:

- Laboratories
- Mechanical rooms
- Operating rooms
- Emergency department
- Clinics and patient rooms
- Facility services and maintenance areas

Loss of environmental support services:

- Heat
- Water supply
- Air-conditioning
- Sterilization
- Electrical power
- Computer network
- Telecommunications (paging, telephones)

Loss of medical gases:

- Oxygen
- Compressed air
- Vacuum suction

Other internal hazards:

- Explosion
- Police actions
- Armed or violent visitor

## External Emergencies and Disasters

Natural hazards:

- Earthquake
- Hurricane
- Flood
- Tornado
- Blizzard

Other external hazards:

- Regional power outage
- Civil disturbance
- Terrorism
- Transportation accidents
- Hazardous materials releases
- Contaminated victims/toxic agents
- Radiation

## Deciding to Evacuate

Orchestrating and successfully completing the task of an orderly evacuation of a hospital or other medical facility is an entirely different process than is recommended for most other buildings and involves special considerations. Because many patients may be medically unstable and/or dependent on mechanical and technology-driven support equipment, complete evacuation of a hospital or other medical facility is to be initiated only as a last resort. The mission of a total evacuation must proceed in a planned and orderly manner. The purpose of the initiation of a plan for total evacuation is to save lives. It is intended to provide for the safety of the health care personnel, facility staff, and patients during a response to an emergency where partial or full patient evacuation may be required.

Evacuation is very difficult to implement. Situations worthy of evacuation include threats posed by fire, smoke, flooding, or a potential exposure to hazardous materials. Evacuation may also be required as a result of structural damage to a facility or the potential for damage imposed by severe changes in climate and/or weather hazards. This is especially true in instances where the dangers to personnel and patients if they remain within the facility are greater than any risks encountered during evacuation. Not all disasters will require an emergency evacuation response. The suggested procedures and considerations listed apply only to those situations when an actual evacuation is necessary.

The decision to initiate an evacuation should be determined by the incident commander (according to the facility's HEICS model). EMS responders are often consulted to assist in determining the need to evacuate a facility. Generally, with most hospital plans, once any consideration is given to implement an evacuation, the medical facility's communications department will be notified so that it can activate internal processes and plans to request the assistance of the applicable public safety personnel. Once a given hospital has activated its plan, a facility's communications department will notify personnel identified in its plans, including public safety and response agencies.

EMS should contact other area hospitals during the response phase if a facility needs to be evacuated. EMS will need information on the emergency room department hospital census, the number of beds available for potential admission, and the number and types of patients the other hospitals can accept. This information will assist the EMS responders in determining their transportation plan and allow the affected hospitals to use their staffs for other assignments such as emergency patient care and movement until EMS arrives.

## How to Evacuate

Dependent upon the severity of the posed threat or hazard, maintaining the patient care and business operations of the hospital/medical facility may require an evacuation. The evacuation of a hospital/medical facility is the most common time that the need for an EMS response would be required. Assisting hospitals and medical facilities should be considered a top priority during EMS preplanning for all potential hazards within an agency's jurisdiction.

During an evacuation of patient care areas, patients should be prioritized for evacuation in the following manner:

1. Patients in immediate danger
2. Ambulatory patients
3. Wheelchairs, isolettes, and cribs
4. Bed-bound patients

Response to a disaster situation should typically be addressed by one or more of the following activities: To defend (shelter) in place, or to conduct a horizontal, vertical, or total evacuation of a medical facility. The concept to defend (shelter) in place is based upon the type of building construction and fire protection systems in the facility. During this tactical maneuver, staff, patients, and visitors may be instructed to remain where they are until further instructions are provided to them. EMS personnel can assist by closing doors and windows in patient rooms, which should provide initial protection from fire. In most incidents, the safest place for patients is in their rooms. Health care providers, including public safety personnel, should never hesitate to relocate because of imminent danger. Certain instructions may be given to maintain order and keep everyone informed of the latest status of the incident. Initiation of a defend (shelter) in place action requires that all routine activities within a medical facility stop, and that preparations are made to enable immediate movement of patients should the incident necessitate such actions as outlined in the following types of patient evacuation.

In a horizontal evacuation, patients are secured from immediate danger but remain on the same floor. Horizontal evacuation typically means that everyone located in the hospital unit in question should be moved to the opposite side of the building, farthest away from the threat or hazard. When a situation escalates, the need for a vertical evacuation may arise.

A vertical evacuation refers to the complete evacuation of a floor, including all units of patient care areas. For a localized incident, occupants can be transferred to an area of refuge identified elsewhere in the hospital, typically at least two floors beneath the incident floor. Generally, areas of refuge are pre-identified in a hospital's evacuation plan in conjunction with any known factors such as hazardous materials storage. In the case of a complete facility evacuation, occupants should be removed to the assigned refuge area. Conscientious efforts should be made by responding personnel to identify, triage, and tag all patients as they leave the floor of origination.

If the tactic of vertical evacuation is unsuccessful, the next course of action is a total evacuation. This stage involves the complete evacuation of the facility. Total evacuation should be initiated only as a last resort. Patients should be transferred to alternate locations and facilities, and sites should be predetermined in the plan. This decision should require coordination between all sections operating under the facility's HEICS. In most instances, the responders from an EMS agency will not be in a position to serve as incident commanders, as this role will be fulfilled by a hospital/medical facility designee, but an EMS responder should be prepared to serve in the capacity for oversight of a treatment, triage, or transportation sector.

Many hospitals formulate mutual aid agreements between other health care facilities within their jurisdiction as part of the planning process to identify sites that can accommodate differing patient populations. For example: Not every medical facility is capable of providing specialized patient care covering needs such as obstetrics, pediatrics, or psychiatry. EMS providers may assist with the hospital's planning efforts to provide guidance regarding the best mechanism to transport these specialized patients and maintain their continuity of care. Some instances may require additional staffing during transportation or an extended care situation, including personnel such as a midwife or respiratory therapist.

> ### EMS and Hospital Preplanning Integration To-Do List
>
> - Identify and list all hospitals and medical facilities within response jurisdiction
> - Identify and make contact with each facility's emergency program manager (or designated planner)
> - Ask for copies of any organizational charts related to the facility and HEICS
> - Share any drafted/created/implemented EMS preplans with each facility's emergency program manager (or designated planner)
> - Ask to view each facility's disaster plan
>   - Including internal/external disaster/emergency plans
> - Inquire of any responses/situations/hazards/threats where the facility presumption is that EMS will be the lead/commander
> - Collaborate to draft facility-specific triage, treatment, and transportation policies and procedures in conjunction with evacuation/shelter-in-place plans
> - Schedule dates to train and exercise the plans together at least once a year
> - Reevaluate, revise EOPs and EMS preplans as
>   - Changes in organizations occur
>   - Disaster/emergency response occurs
> - Implement best practices/lessons learned from any similar hazard/threat responses identified in EOPs or EMS preplans (Example: Jurisdiction may not have been affected by recent flu outbreak, but plans can be modified from others' experiences)

## Selected References

Adini, R, Goldberg, A, et al.: Assessing levels of hospital emergency preparedness. *Prehosp Disaster Med* 2006;21(6):451–457.

Committee on the Future of Emergency Care in the United States Health System: *Hospital-Based Emergency Care: At the Breaking Point.* Washington, D.C.: The National Academies Press; 2007.

FEMA: *Guide for All Hazards Planning Emergency Operations Planning.* Washington D.C.: FEMA; September, 1996.

Freyberg, C, Arquilla, B, et al.: Disaster preparedness: Hospital decontamination and the pediatric patient—Guidelines for hospitals and emergency planners. *Prehosp Disaster Med* 2008;23(2):166–172.

Gildea, J and Etengoff, S: Vertical evacuation simulation of critically ill patients in a hospital. *Prehosp Disaster Med* 2005;20(4):243–248.

Grentenkort, P, Harke, H, et al.: Interface between hospital and fire authorities: A concept for management of incidents in hospitals. *Prehosp Disaster Med* 2002;17(1):42–47.

Hamilton, DR, Gavagan, TF, et al.: Houston's medical disaster response to Hurricane Katrina: Part 1, The initial medical response from trauma service area Q. *Ann Emerg Med* 2009;53(4):505–514.

Hamilton, DR, Gavagan, TF, et al.: Houston's medical disaster response to Hurricane Katrina: Part 2, transitioning from emergency evacuee care to community health care. *Ann Emerg Med* 2009;53(4):515–527.

Hersche, B and Wenker, O: Principles of hospital disaster planning. *The Internet Journal of Rescue and Disaster Medicine* 2003; 1(2).

Hsu, EB, Jenckes, MW, et al.: *Training of Hospital Staff to Respond To A Mass Casualty Incident. Evidence Report/ Technology Assessment: Number 95.* Rockville, MD: Agency for Healthcare Research and Quality; April, 2004.

Hsu, E, Grabowski, J, et al.: Effects of local emergency departments of large scale urban chemical fire with hazardous materials spill. *Prehosp Disaster Med* 2002;17(4):196–201.

Hsu, E, Jenckes, M, et al.: Effectiveness of hospital staff mass-casualty incident training methods: A systematic literature review. *Prehosp Disaster Med* 2004;19(3):191–199.

Kanter, R, Andrake, J, et al.: Developing consensus on appropriate standards of disaster care for children. *Disaster Med Public Health Prep* 2009;3(1):5–7.

Kuba, M, Dorian, A, et al.: *Elderly Populations in Disasters: Recounting Evacuation Processes from Two Skilled-Care Facilities in Florida,* UCLA Center for Public Health and Disasters; August, 2004.

Levinson, DR *Nursing Home Emergency Preparedness and Response During Recent Hurricanes.* Washington, D.C.: Department of Health and Human Services, Office of Inspector General; August, 2006.

Mohammed, A, Mann, H, et al.: Impact of London's terrorist attacks on a major trauma center in London. *Prehosp Disaster Med* 2006;21(5):340–344.

O'Sullivan, T, Amaratunga, C, et al.: If schools are closed, who will watch our kids? Family caregiving and other sources of role conflict among nurses during large scale outbreaks. *Prehosp Disaster Med* 2009;24(4):321–325.

Pan-American Health Organization, Regional Office, World Health Organization: *Hospitals in Disasters: Handle with Care Discussion Guide*; July, 2003.

Rubin, J: *Recurring Pitfalls in Hospital Preparedness and Response.* http://www.homelandsecurity.org; January, 2004. Accessed August 28, 2007.

Schultz, C, Koenig, K, et al.: Benchmarking for hospital evacuation: A critical data collection tool. *Prehosp Disaster Med* 2005;20(5):331–342.

Stenberg, E, Lee, G, et al.: Counting crises: US hospital evacuations 1971–1999. *Prehosp Disaster Med* 2004;19(2):150–157.

Taaffee, K, Kohl, R, et al.: *Hospital Evacuation: Issues and Complexities Proceeding of the 2005 Winter Simulation Conference.* Clemson, SC: Clemson University; 2005.

Thorne, C, Levitin, H, et al.: A pilot assessment of hospital preparedness for bioterrorism events. *Prehosp Disaster Med* 2006;21(6):414–422.

Tokuda, Y, Kikuchi, M, et al.: Pre-hospital management of sarin nerve gas terrorism in urban settings: 10 years of progress after the Tokyo subway sarin attack. *Resuscitation* 2006;68(2):193–202.

Treat, K, Williams, J, et al.: Hospital preparedness for weapons of mass destruction incidents: An initial assessment. *Ann Emerg Med* 2001;38(5):562–565.

United States Fire Administration: Topical fire research series. *Medical Facility Fires* 2002; 2(8).

Zane, R and Prestipino, A: Implementing the hospital emergency incident command system: An integrated delivery system's experience. *Prehosp Disaster Med* 2004;19(4):311–317.

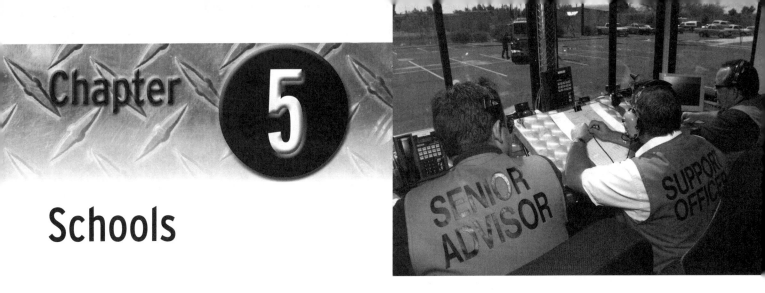

# Chapter 5

# Schools

## Introduction to Preplanning for Schools

On October 2, 2006, a 32-year-old truck driver attacked the West Nickel Mines School, a one-room Amish school in Lancaster County, PA. Eleven girls were shot, and five of them were killed. Such a tragedy can cause an entire community to mourn, affect the emotional health of responders, and significantly impact normal operations of the school system; an entire replacement school was built for West Nickel Mines.

Emergencies at schools can evoke strong emotional reactions because of the community's ties to the school and the impact on children and adolescents. A serious incident at an elementary school evokes tremendous outpouring of emotion from parents and the community at large. This makes effective management of the scene difficult. While adequate preplanning can never decrease the emotional response to these incidents, through planning and training, emergency medical services (EMS) providers may respond in an efficient and orderly fashion. This is a major reason to preplan for these types of events; preplanning provides a mechanism for defining a strategy and identifying resources to lessen the effects on both rescuers and the community. The following case studies illustrate the need for EMS preplanning in schools.

### Case Studies

#### Columbine High School

High school seniors Dylan Klebold and Eric Harris assaulted Columbine High School in Littleton, CO, in an attempt to murder hundreds of students and school staff on April 20, 1999. Twelve students and one teacher were killed, and many others were injured before Klebold and Harris shot themselves in their heads. The two used a semiautomatic handgun, rifle, shotguns, and multiple small bombs in the attack after two propane bombs they had planted in the school cafeteria failed to detonate. According to evidence found in the Klebold and Harris homes, initial planning for a "massacre" began a year before the attack, and Klebold had contemplated suicide as early as 1997.

#### West Nickel Mines School

On October 2, 2006, a truck driver attacked a one-room Amish schoolhouse, the West Nickel Mines School in Lancaster County, PA. Twenty-six students aged 6 to 13 were at the school. Thirty-two-year-old Charlie Roberts allowed the boys and teacher to go free, then shot eleven girls execution style, killing five and

*continues*

critically wounding six others before shooting himself. Roberts had three children of his own, was not previously wanted by the authorities, and had no criminal record.

### Virginia Tech

On April 16, 2007, Virginia Tech student Cho Seung-Hui killed 33 people and injured many more as he went door to door in a dormitory and then a classroom building on the campus of Virginia Tech in Blacksburg, VA. Cho used two handguns to shoot his victims before he took his own life with a gunshot to the head. Police investigated Cho twice in the fall of 2005 after receiving complaints from women about harassment. A Virginia judge declared Cho an "imminent danger to himself because of mental illness" and ordered outpatient psychiatric treatment in 2005.

Schools should be considered distinct and separate entities from other facilities due to their unique populations and issues. They may include preschools, primary/elementary, middle, and high schools; junior and four-year colleges; technical and vocational schools; as well as fire, police, or public safety training academies. A community may have anywhere from one to several school facilities, both private and public. Many public educational facilities provide some level of programs for children with special needs, medical special needs persons, children with disciplinary problems, or severe handicaps. These special populations must be considered in order to preplan effectively for schools.

In preplanning for educational facilities, it is important to determine what challenges are present at the facility. Although some are similar, there are distinct differences between educational facilities that would present unique challenges to EMS. For example, medical special needs is a term that describes persons dependent on medical technology in order to live or function, and may present immediate patient care concerns such as ventilators, medication pumps, or even special wheelchairs for mobility (see **Figure 5-1**). In contrast, the term special needs children describes children who need some form of assistance but may not have a potential for immediate patient care concern. They are still a significant consideration during preplanning and response. Examples would include emotionally challenged children, mobility impaired children, or children who are blind or deaf.

Natural disasters such as hurricanes and tornadoes, fires, geographic-specific emergencies such as flooding and earthquakes, and large crowds present for sporting events, recitals, plays, and other special events make preplanning for schools crucial. Unfortunately, deadly, large-scale shooting events such as Columbine and Virginia Tech necessitate planning as well.

While this chapter addresses the basic planning steps for all types of schools including colleges and universities, it is important to consider how childhood development and cognitive ability may impact a response to a kindergarten, elementary, or middle school. Younger children may be very dependent on routine and the presence of teachers and staff to guide them through daily functions. Large-scale emergencies can result in confusion and separation from the child's usual guide.

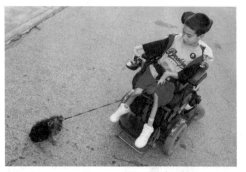

**Figure 5-1** EMS agencies should consider what resources are required to provide care for medical special needs children when preplanning for schools.

## Childhood Development and Cognitive Abilities

Children aged 3 to 6 years begin to have an intuitive grasp on some logical concepts, but concepts that are formed tend to be very simple—and irreversible. At this stage of cognitive development, events are easily explained as "magical." The child's perceptions dominate his or her judgment, and reality is not firm.

During the ages of 6 to 12 years, children become capable of organized, logical thought. Thinking becomes less egocentric, and the child is capable of concrete problem solving.

As adolescence begins during the ages of 12 to 18 years, children are able to incorporate formal logic into thought. They can generate multiple hypotheses, estimate outcomes, and think more abstractly. **Table 5-1** outlines the cognitive abilities associated with each age group.

| **Table 5-1** Cognitive Development in Children | |
|---|---|
| **Age** | **Cognitive Abilities** |
| 3 to 6 years | Intuitive grasp on simple concepts; children's own perceptions dominate their judgment. |
| 6 to 12 years | Capable of organized, logical thought and concrete problem solving; less egocentric. |
| 12 to 18 years | Incorporate formal logic into thought; capable of estimating outcomes (deduction) and thinking abstractly. |

Although much of the discussion has been and will concentrate on schools designed for younger populations, such as elementary schools, the concepts described can be incorporated relatively easily when considering a college or university setting. The biggest difference lies in the cognitive abilities of the students and scope, or size, of the facility.

## Planning for Emergencies Within the School

An American Academy of Pediatrics survey in 2004 asked school principals and superintendents about their preparedness activities for mass-casualty/terrorism events. Eighty-three percent of respondents indicated that they had response plans. Ninety-five percent of schools indicated that they had an evacuation plan to move students from the school in case of a terrorist event either on foot, by bus, via parents, or other means. Thirty percent of respondents with an evacuation plan had never exercised it. Twenty-two percent had no provisions within their response plans for children with special health care needs or mobility concerns. Some schools (42.8%) indicated they had never met with EMS services to discuss emergency planning.

Remember "Learn Not to Burn" and "Stop, Drop, and Roll"? The American fire service has been incredibly proactive and effective in reaching school-age children with its fire prevention messages. School accreditation standards and state and local fire codes mandate periodic fire inspections and fire drills for school facilities, but the fire service has taken its responsibilities for life safety inspections and drills a step further by developing relationships with school officials to take advantage of the captive audiences found in elementary schools to deliver educational messages that students enjoy and take home with them. By the third grade, every student in the country has drawn a home fire escape plan and has taken it home to conduct a fire drill with mom and dad.

EMS can deliver its public education message to this same audience and develop its own facility preplans. Public educators and planners will likely find the same cooperation from school systems that the fire service has if EMS simply asks. EMS administrators must program an adequate budget and personnel time for planning activities and appoint EMS liaison officers and planners to work with local schools.

### School Nurses

School nurses are vital during student health emergencies and can be a significant resource for EMS both during preplanning and actual emergencies. Although not all school systems utilize school nurses, each school system has someone designated to fulfill the essential functions of the school nurse. This person is charged with evaluating student health and notifying parents of illness or injury. Even schools that do have school nurse coverage may not have nurse coverage during the entire school day. Based on school location, school system size, budget constraints, and other factors, a single nurse may rotate among several schools during the day. In those models with limited nursing coverage, other key individuals, usually administrators, may be assigned to manage medical emergencies and minor illnesses in the nurse's absence.

According to Olympia, Wan, and Avner, school nurses self-reported more confidence in managing respiratory distress, airway obstruction, bleeding, fractures, anaphylaxis, and diabetic emergencies in a 2005 survey. School nurses reported less confidence with cardiac arrest, overdose, seizures, heat-related illness, and head injury. While head injuries and seizures account for two of the five most reported school medical emergencies, the survey indicates that roughly half of school nurses self report confidence handling these cases. This may be another rapport-building opportunity for EMS. Why not invite the local school nurses association to your agency's continuing education classes or even jointly sponsor a school- and/or community-wide cardiopulmonary resuscitation (CPR) program? The EMS agency training officer may be able to obtain continuing medical education (CME) certification so that nurses can be awarded CME credit or assist school nurses to maintain professional certification. EMS agencies can also help by assisting with training exercises and simulations for school nurses and other staff members.

The Olympia, Wan, and Avner study shows that most respondents had been nurses for over 5 years, and that the two most common medical complaints they managed were sprains and shortness of breath. Sixty-eight percent of nurses reported they had managed an emergency for which EMS had been called within the past year. Eighty-six percent of respondents indicated that their school had a medical emergency response plan (MERP) as suggested by the American Academy of Pediatrics and the American Heart Association (AHA), but 35% of those schools did not practice the plan, and 13% of schools did not identify authorized personnel to make emergency medical decisions for minor children in the event of an emergency.

Regulations governing age of consent for medical decision making vary from state to state. An important element for the EMS preplan for schools will be identification of those responsible for medical decision making in the absence of parents. Seventeen percent or more of schools may not have an authorized, designated staff member responsible for medical decision making. This designation should be a part of the school's MERP, and it should be captured in the EMS preplan. Additionally, EMS providers should maintain familiarity with regulations and protocols in their state that provide guidance on consent issues.

The AHA's scientific statement on MERPS recommends medical emergency simulation training for school staff and also provides a recommended list of emergency supplies and equipment including automatic defibrillators, epinephrine, oxygen, and glucagon. It is recommended that schools provide a copy of their MERP to local responders. EMS agencies can assist schools in creating their plan by educating school staff on the local emergency response system, capabilities of EMS, local medical protocols, and conducting exercises and medical emergency simulations.

## Medical Emergency Response Plan for Schools

Medical Emergency Response Plan for Schools (MERPS) is a public health project coordinated by the AHA to help schools respond to medical emergencies in the first few minutes before the arrival of EMS. The AHA provides written guidance on how to develop and maintain a coordinated and practiced response plan. Critical elements of an MERP are:

- Effective and efficient communication throughout the school campus
- Coordinated and practiced response plan
- Risk reduction
- Training and equipment for first aid and CPR
- Implementation of a lay rescuer automated external defibrillator (AED) program

## Student Medications

In many school systems, students are required to keep all medications with the school nurse or administrators; many school systems do not allow students to have possession of Epi-Pens or even over-the-counter pain relievers. An important element of the EMS preplan will be the identification of the school employee with access to health records, medication lists, or other alerts concerning students with chronic medical conditions and the location of and access to students' medications.

## Planning Issues

Schools are unique in the variability of their populations, activities and operations, and special circumstances. One of the best ways to ensure that all factors are evaluated during preplanning is to take an organized approach to the planning process. The planning process can be broken down into three main, overlapping phases: estimating the incident and collecting data.

> ### Preplanning for Schools—Definition
>
> **In loco parentis:** Latin for "in place of a parent." Based in English common law, the legal doctrine that refers to a person or institution that assumes parental rights and duties for a minor. The most frequent usage of in loco parentis relates to teachers and their students.

### Estimation of the Incident

One of the first steps in developing the preplan is to ask the question "what is being planned for?" Planners must make an educated estimate about the worst-case scenario and plan for that scenario according to the planner's and organization's capabilities and resources available. Perhaps even more important is to plan for what is the most likely scenario. To imagine either scenario, the planner must collect and evaluate facts and make assumptions.

Facts include all of the data collected during preplanning visits, interviews and discussions with school officials, information available from government sources, and consultation with partner response agencies such as police, fire, and emergency management officials. Assumptions include educated predictions of population behavior, estimates of the likelihood of occurrences, and possible variations in emergency response. For example, a simplified collection of facts and assumptions about "Your Town Primary School" might look like this:

*Facts:*

- Your Town Primary is located in a rural area, approximately 6 miles from the county's main, four-lane highway.
- There is a railroad track one third of a mile from the school highly utilized for freight shipments.
- Daily student load is 208 students aged 6 to 13 years.
- There are three students with significant vision or hearing impairment.
- There is one student with an implanted vagal nerve stimulation device (due to a severe seizure disorder).
- There are no students or staff with limited mobility.
- Daily full-time staffing includes 21 teachers, administrators, and support staff.
- The only hazardous material on the grounds is a 150-gallon gasoline tank used for fueling lawn maintenance equipment.
- The current Your Town Primary was constructed 4 years ago, replacing a much older facility just down the road.
- There is no full-time, assigned security officer or school resource officer.
- Local fire and EMS are all volunteer, with two ambulances available if the crew is paged out.
- Closest mutual aid ambulance support is a neighboring community 15 minutes away.

*Assumptions:*

- School staff will have to handle the first 10 to 20 minutes of any medical emergency.
- A serious fire is unlikely due to the building's modern, fire-resistant construction.

- Mass-casualty situations would most likely result from a natural disaster, gas leak or explosion, or fire- or hazardous materials–related transportation accident on the nearby railroad.
- Transportation of a large number of wounded children would be delayed due to the rural character of the area and limited EMS resources.
- Alternative EMS transport and extensive mutual aid will be required for any large incident.
- The population of students and staff should be able to effectively self-evacuate from the building as long as no significant structural damage is caused by an incident.
- There is adequate staff to assist and supervise the student population, including a low number of students with disabilities.
- Any mass-casualty incident (MCI) would likely occur during school hours.

When an EMS planner analyzes the facts and assumptions for Your Town Primary, the estimation may look like this:

- The incident most likely to occur would be a routine medical emergency.
- The worst-case scenario would be an MCI resulting from a natural disaster, natural gas emergency, or rail accident involving hazardous materials with the potential for up to 229 victims (not including any school visitors).

Before planning a response, EMS must collect solid facts on the facility in question, make assumptions, analyze the data and assumptions, and estimate the type of response required.

## Data Collection

Preplanning an EMS incident at a school should mirror the process fire departments use for preplanning. The data collected should be accurate, organized, and recorded in the preplan document. The most basic data involves the actual facility and its population, so the best place to start is with a visit to the school to meet with administrators and tour the facility.

Whether EMS starts with an informal contact with a school representative or more formal written correspondence such as a letter or email, they should set an appointment. EMS should plan on meeting for 30 to 60 minutes. At this appointment, EMS can explain the planning process, the importance of a preplan for the crews, and collect basic facility and demographic information. They should also speak with the school nurse, any security or resource officer, and maintenance or custodial staff that are familiar with the buildings and grounds. EMS should ask for a building diagram if it is not available from the fire department or not already incorporated into the dispatch system and available digitally on a mobile data terminal in response vehicles.

Depending on time spent in the initial meeting, the rapport developed with school staff, and information already available from other sources, EMS may need to ask for an additional appointment to tour the facility (and possibly even sketch a diagram, if one is not available). A tour and familiarization may take anywhere from less than an hour to several days, depending on the size and complexity of the building and campus, and the availability of existing diagrams, site plans, or blueprints.

### Preplanning Practices

Fire inspectors do not show up unannounced for routine inspections and neither should EMS. The school administrator's time is valuable, and it is important to establish a good rapport in order to receive maximum cooperation with the planning process. Any time the administrator is spending with EMS is most likely time that would be spent providing instruction, meeting with staff, parents, or students, or other administrative or supervisory tasks. EMS has much to offer the school in public education opportunities, assistance with drills and exercises, and expert consultation and training on managing medical emergencies, automatic defibrillation programs, and other areas. The school staff has a wealth of information that EMS needs in order to effectively plan. Both EMS and the school will benefit from a well-planned, coordinated response to an emergency.

To streamline the visit and efficiently use time on site at the school, EMS should contact and collaborate with other local government agencies before the appointment. It is important to review the fire department's preplan and speak with the inspector or fire marshal that normally inspects the school. If not included in the fire department's preplan, the municipal planning or zoning office should be able to provide building diagrams and site plans. EMS can ask the emergency communications center for an address history on the school from the computer-aided dispatch (CAD) system. The address history will show the number of fire, EMS, and/or police responses to an address and the time of day those calls occurred over a given period of time.

### Daily Census and Student Demographics

How many students are likely to be in the building on any given school day? The total number of possible patients for an MCI will help EMS planners in creating predetermined alarm box assignments for certain types of alarms. In the Your Town Primary example, only two ambulances are typically available. So in planning for an MCI, it would be prudent to have a predetermined dispatch box that results in the needed mutual aid resources automatically being alerted and dispatched. This type of resource bundling or "box" for a special incident or MCI at Your Town Primary would need to include ambulances, supervisors, and support equipment from neighboring communities, private ambulance services, and other available resources.

While EMS staff and transport resources are the most visible and versatile resources, the census also can assist in planning for the medical supplies and equipment that would be needed for mass-casualty medical care. With the transport resources available, it is likely that a significant number of lower-acuity patients would remain on scene for some time before transport was available. Equipment and consumable supplies such as backboards, soft goods like bandages and dressings, oxygen equipment, blankets, and other supplies can be stored on vehicles and trailers or pre-staged in or near the facility. The number of potential patients can help drive the assembly of a realistic supply cache.

Student demographics and characteristics are also important in creating a preconfigured dispatch plan. A school with a large number of very young or disabled students such as mentally challenged students or persons with significant mobility challenges would dictate more manpower on the initial alarm assignment, since such a population would be less able to adequately respond to an MCI. This type of population would also require more staff in the holding or medical treatment area for supervision.

Initial planning information for Your Town Primary indicates that one student has a history of frequent seizures and has an implanted vagal nerve stimulation device. Most student populations will have some students with special medical needs. Since the routine medical emergency is likely to be the most frequent call for service to any school, it is important that EMS providers are familiar with any special conditions or medical equipment that may be encountered. During the preplanning process, students with special needs can be identified by school administration or the school nurse. EMS agencies and the EMS medical director should evaluate existing protocols and policies to ensure that EMS providers have the necessary training and scope of practice to provide a satisfactory level of care to these students.

As was mentioned earlier, students with special needs may use medical equipment or implanted devices such as a vagal nerve stimulators, tracheostomy tubes, cerebrospinal fluid shunts, or other devices. Students with mobility problems may have special wheelchairs or other equipment. Children with chronic conditions may also have prescribed medications available at the school, including diazepam gel for rectal administration, medications for allergies and breathing problems, insulin, and others. Schools should maintain an emergency information form (EIF) for children with chronic conditions and special health care needs (see **Figure 5-2**); the custodian of the EIF forms would normally be the school nurse, and should be identified in the EMS preplan. The EIF is a standardized form containing a child's medical history, medications, special contact information, and suggested initial treatment. The EIF is filled out by the child's parents or physician and can be invaluable to EMS providers and health care providers at the definitive care facility where the child is ultimately transported.

Students with communication or sensory disabilities such as deafness, blindness, or speech problems can be challenging for EMS providers who have had no exposure to these conditions. Mechanisms to ensure that EMS can communicate with these students should be identified and noted in the preplan and can range from training some EMS providers in American Sign Language to identifying staff or other students who can be transported along with the patient to act as an interpreter.

School Year 20__

## Medical Emergency and Special Needs

Information provided on this form is voluntary. This form is intended for children with chronic medical conditions. Completion of this form is not legally binding, but the information provided will be used for planning purposes if your child has a medical emergency. It will not be used for any other purpose. The information will be maintained for one year from the start of the school year. Please complete the form and return it to your child's school.

Student's Name: _____ Date of Birth: ___/___/_____
Address: _____
School: _____ Grade: _____
Medical History: (eg, asthma, diabetes, heart condition, cancer, etc.)
_____
_____
Medication Allergies: Y___ N ___ *If yes, please list:* _____
Special Health Care Needs: (eg, ventilator, heart monitor, oxygen, wheelchair, etc.)
_____
_____
Special Equipment Needed: Y___ N ___ *If yes, please list:* _____
Physician: _____ Telephone: _____
Additional Information: _____
_____

**Parent Contact Information:**
Name: _____ Telephone: (____) ____-_____
Alternate Contact Person/Information:
Name: _____ Telephone: _____
Signature: _____ Date: ___/___/_____

Fax to (XXX) XXX-XXXX
                    Fire Department Use
_____
Stations
Home: _____    School: _____

**Figure 5-2** Emergency information forms are an important source of information concerning the special needs of students.

### Time/Season of Incident

While it may not be feasible to plan or create dispatch boxes for different times of the day or school year, it is important for planners and EMS supervisors to be aware that the student-to-teacher ratio may vary based on the type of school event and season. For instance, there may be many more students per each adult staff member for after school sports practice. During assemblies or sporting events there will be many students in one place. These type of events also have many parents and other adults in attendance. During a school evacuation or fire drill during the school day, administrators and teachers normally have a predetermined method of accounting for each student after the evacuation, and reporting that accountability to the principal or other administrator. During a special event during the evening such as a play or recital, this normal accountability process will likely not be used since students may not be grouped with their normal classmates and teachers. The accountability process outside regular school hours should be considered by the incident commander and EMS supervisor and may result in a more aggressive interior search for certain incident types, or more fire, EMS, and police personnel may be needed on the scene to manage and direct the evacuees.

Summer school and other summer events also may result in a larger student-to-teacher ratio, since the school day is normally shorter, and many assistants and other school support staff are not employed outside the regular school year.

### Facility and Physical Plant and Grounds

The preplan document should indicate where the EMS crew should report and specify that a school staff member meet EMS to guide them to the location of the emergency. If the reporting location is different during a school lockdown or other special circumstance, this also should be identified and listed in the preplan document.

Advance planning goes a long way to avoid scene chaos by predesignating staging areas for various types of equipment. EMS should consult with the fire department and other response agencies regarding what their predicted apparatus set up plan would be for various events (fires, bomb threats, MCIs). The school grounds can be scouted in advance for areas that would make the preferred "treatment" areas for a mass-casualty situation. Ideally, this area will have close proximity to a paved road or parking lot where ambulances can stage, then be called up to receive patients and depart without creating traffic jams.

Secondary staging areas also should be indicated in the preplan. For a large incident utilizing many ambulances, buses, and other methods of transport, or a scene with limited operating space, a secondary staging area is the collection point for all transport resources initially arriving on scene. These resources are identified and categorized by the staging officer, then sent up to the primary staging area as needed and as space allows. A secondary staging area may be a few blocks up to a mile or more away from the scene. Ideal secondary staging areas, such as church and shopping center parking lots, nearby fire stations, or other government buildings, are easily identified by mutual aid responders who may not be familiar with the location.

It may not be feasible for a school staff member to meet EMS at a central or predesignated location at facilities with multiple buildings or a large campus. For this type of facility, it is especially important that building diagrams and site plans or maps be included in the EMS preplan document for responders. During planning visits, EMS planners should note how emergency communications would occur within the school, and whether each classroom and building has an emergency bill. A "fire bill" or "emergency bill" is a sign near the door of each classroom that should identify the room's maximum occupancy, emergency telephone number, specific address, and building or room numbers/specific location within that address.

Emergency shelters, if present, should be noted in the preplan document and indicated on the building or site diagrams. Fallout shelters exist in many older government buildings including schools. These fallout shelters were designed during the Cold War to provide shelter against radiological fallout or radiological particles after a nuclear blast during a nuclear exchange with the Soviet Union.

School buildings in certain parts of the country may be equipped with tornado or storm shelters. Knowledge of shelter locations and capabilities are important for emergency services since some emergencies such as fire or building collapse will necessitate that the building be searched. In other incidents, EMS may be responding to a school to treat an adult from the community who sought protection in a shelter due to a weather event or other natural disaster. Community members who rapidly sought shelter may have left their homes without required prescription medications or other medical supplies and written medical history information.

## Security Situations and Planning

Based on the school's planning and site layout, security incidents may impact the EMS preplan. It has already been noted that a lockdown situation may change the location where the ambulances report for a medical emergency, but law enforcement contingency plans for shootings, hostage situations, and bomb threats may designate certain standoff distances or access requirements that also affect preplanned medical treatment and staging areas. Just as EMS must coordinate with the fire department for preplanning the incident scene for noncriminal events, local law enforcement should be consulted for assistance with preplanning the EMS response to criminal events.

Evening events at school facilities may also affect the EMS report location and staging. A show or assembly in an auditorium, gym, or cafeteria may result in the attendees being some distance away from the entrance usually used by EMS during the school day. Additionally, many building entrances and exits may be locked at night.

School resource officers (SROs) can be a valuable asset during emergencies. The SRO serves as a visible law enforcement presence on school property to respond to emergencies and deter and prevent crime. SROs may be affiliated with local or state police, sheriff's departments, or private security firms. Most are actually sworn personnel with police powers. SROs also may serve as informal advisors to students or conflict resolution specialists. The presence or absence of an SRO is valuable information to have in the EMS preplan when responding to calls that would normally cause the EMS crew to stop and wait for law enforcement arrival prior to proceeding to the scene (such as assaults and gun and knife wounds). SROs should be incorporated into preplanning along with school administrators and nurses due to their insight on law enforcement–related contingencies such as security plans, the specifics of lockdown procedures, and building access.

Another important preplanning aspect of police and security at schools is the designation of a law enforcement representative for the command post. Any large or prolonged incident at a school will most likely result in a unified command involving fire, EMS, and the school division. A criminal or terrorist incident will necessitate adding law enforcement to the unified command: law enforcement will have primary command and tactical control during a criminal or terrorist incident.

## Special Hazards

School facilities may include specialty education areas that contain some quantity of hazardous materials. Examples include biology, chemistry, and physics labs, and vocational or trade school offerings such as auto mechanics and heating and air-conditioning repair. Hazardous materials may range from small amounts of chemicals used in labs to large, pressurized gas cylinders. College and university science labs may host larger and more varied quantities of chemical substances. Some advance knowledge of hazardous materials storage locations is important to EMS for two reasons: Personal safety for the EMS crews and the possibility of treating injuries resulting from chemical exposure.

During preplanning site visits, EMS planners should inquire about the use and storage of hazardous materials. These should be noted on the preplan along with the type of storage container, quantity, and location. An important resource for EMS providers during a chemical emergency will be the material safety data sheet (MSDS). Each hazardous chemical will have its own MSDS that lists specific decontamination steps, personal protective equipment recommended for responders, and a guide to medical treatment. The Occupational Health and Safety Administration's Hazard Communication Standard requires that employers maintain MSDS for hazardous chemicals used in their workplaces. Ideally, the MSDS will be stored in a central location that is easily accessed by employees and responders. The location of the facility's MSDS library should be noted on the EMS preplan.

Specific antidotes are recommended for certain dangerous chemicals. EMS planners should collaborate with school system or college lab directors, the fire department, hazardous materials team, and medical direction to determine the feasibility of maintaining specific treatments and antidotes that may lie outside normal EMS protocols. Universities and industries that work with certain hazardous substances may already keep antidotes on hand; in this instance, it is important that EMS be aware of the antidote's availability and maintain familiarity with its administration.

Earlier in the chapter while discussing facts and assumptions for Your Town Primary School, it was noted that a busy railroad line used mostly for freight transportation was located approximately one third of a mile from the school. While estimating the potential for large-scale emergencies at a school facility it is important to include possible transportation or industrial emergencies that may occur close to the school as a source for a mass-casualty or large-scale evacuation. EMS planners should attempt to identify petroleum or chemical pipelines, major industries such as fuel refineries and gas distribution centers, railroads and major highways where large containers of hazardous materials are transported, and other hazards.

EMS planners should ensure that preplanning for a specific facility does not conflict with existing plans for industrial and transportation emergencies that already exist in the jurisdiction. In many cases, sheltering and evacuation plans for large-scale industrial and transportation incidents may already be a part of the jurisdiction's local emergency plan. Two excellent sources for this information will be the locality's emergency manager and the local emergency planning committee (LEPC).

LEPCs are links between industry, government, and citizens with the goal of enhancing hazardous materials emergency preparedness. Many LEPCs go further and are also involved with all-hazards emergency plans. Large-scale transportation or industrial incidents may impact response and evacuation routes, sites for treatment and transportation, and predetermined staging areas.

## Other Considerations

Other issues to consider while preplanning for schools include the possibility of involving key school staff personnel in some manner in the incident command system (ICS). An EMS agency may decide to utilize school staff within the medical branch of an incident, for a communications strategy, or for help with public affairs and working with the media.

### School Staff and the ICS

A unified command, versus a single incident commander, will likely be the most effective incident command model at any prolonged incident involving a school. Other than fire, police, and EMS, other primary stakeholders in a school-related incident will be the local school system and possibly the municipal emergency manager. Fire and EMS, and increasingly emergency management staff, are well practiced with utilizing ICS. School system representatives may be less familiar and practiced with ICS, which presents an opportunity for EMS to further develop its relationship with the local school system. The EMS agency in conjunction with other local emergency response agencies or the local emergency manager can steer school system administrators to the basic, online National Incident Management System (NIMS) courses. Integration of principals and school system superintendents or other senior staff in unified command should be practiced in exercises.

A method of credentialing or identification should also be considered (How does EMS know that this person is really the assistant superintendent of schools?). One possibility is the use of identification vests similar to those used by fire and EMS could also be acquired by the school system and available for emergencies. School officials and local response agencies can collaborate on color coding and titles ("principal," "school transportation," "school liaison") for the school's ICS vests so that the school officials can be identified but not confuse responders.

> ### Local Emergency Planning Committee
>
> Title III of the Superfund Amendments and Reauthorization Act of 1986, also known as the Federal Emergency Planning and Community Right-To-Know Act established responsibilities for hazardous chemical emergency planning, among other requirements for businesses and federal, state, and local governments. LEPCs were established as planning entities, and a link between industry, citizens, and government in the wake of the Bhopal, India chemical disaster. On December 3, 1984, 42 tons of methyl isocyanate, a cyanide gas, was released from a Union Carbide pesticide plant, killing almost 4,000 people. Subsequent investigation determined that the release was most likely caused by intentional sabotage.

## School Staff in the MCI Medical Branch

In addition to involving school system employees at the command level of incident management, EMS planners should consider involving certain key school personnel in the medical branch. The school nurse could assist in the secondary triage area or treatment group. After initial triage and movement to the treatment area, the school nurse may be very helpful in identifying students with underlying chronic medical conditions or special needs that might impact their treatment and transport priority.

While crucial at all mass-casualty events, accountability of patients will be a high priority at events involving school-aged children. A school administrator, secretary, or teachers may be able to assist the transportation officer and transportation recorder with accurately identifying children and logging their destination as they are moved to transportation resources and taken for medical treatment.

## Communication Strategy

There is normally intense media interest in large emergencies, and particularly so for violent criminal events such as shootings or other terrorist-style attacks. During more routine emergencies such as house fires or automobile accidents, fire and EMS agencies normally utilize an agency public information officer as the designated spokesperson to deliver press releases and entertain questions from media. On a large-scale, unified command incident, it is critical to maintain unity of public information as well as unity of command. This unity of message can be accomplished with an overall communication strategy.

The communication strategy is a planned approach to disseminating information regarding a particular incident or type of incident. The major components of a communication strategy include background information and overall objectives of the strategy that include key messages, specific methods of information dissemination, and evaluation of the strategy.

The background information may include key points of the EMS agency and other responders, the location of the incident, and the type of facility or incident type. Additionally, background may explain if any specific training for such an incident or facility has been undertaken.

The overall purpose or objective of the communication strategy is to identify potential audiences, such as the public, or possibly families in the case of school incidents. Additionally, key messages can be drafted as part of the preplanning process to address basic issues. Many prepared messages for various issues can be obtained from the Centers for Disease Control or prepared locally. These prepared messages are designed to meet the need of the media to have and disseminate information during the initial stages of an incident and also buy time while the situation evolves. Information is delivered and can be effective in delaying the media from "freelancing" around the incident looking for newsworthy tidbits.

Besides looking at the primary audience, such as the public, and the secondary audience, such as the families of children involved, the communication strategy also should address how messages are released from the EMS agency. This involves coordinating how information about an incident will be released through print media, traditional radio, television, as well as online media.

The final and key aspect of the communication strategy is the evaluation of the strategy. Even if the EMS agency does not have a specific local incident to evaluate, evaluation can be done by examining media coverage of other events around the world. What common and even peculiar elements are present, and how do those elements impact the EMS organization's strategy utilizing the same media?

## Media and Public Affairs

It is imperative that the message delivered to the public via the media be accurate and consistent, particularly when it concerns injured or deceased students. Utilizing multiple, independent spokespersons from the school system, police, fire, EMS, and the municipality will increase the chances of multiple variations in information released, and result in an inconsistent message. For these reasons a joint information center (JIC) should be established to advise the unified command on public affairs issues related to the response and to deliver information and press releases to the media. The JIC structure works within the framework of the ICS. The information officer (IO) is appointed by the incident commander/unified command and has the responsibility of initial organization of the JIC and management of JIC operations. The JIC is composed of representatives of the agencies involved in the response and has three primary responsibilities:

1. Collect information about the incident
2. Analyze public perceptions of the response
3. Deliver information to the public

Like the ICS, the JIC is modular and flexible and may grow as large as the incident dictates with its own branches and divisions and support staff for the IO. The JIC serves as the centralized information hub responsible for delivering efficient, consistent communications to the public.

## Parental Notification

EMS planners should review the school's MERP during preplanning meetings and note whether there is a mechanism in place for mass notification of many parents. Some school systems may use automatic phone message systems, group emails, or text messages for this purpose. Whatever the method, it should be identified in the school's emergency plan. Ideally there will also be a backup plan (such as transfer of this function to the school division offices) in the event of structural damage to the school building.

## Incidents Involving School Buses

An emergency involving a school bus may be considered a remote, smaller version of an incident that occurs at a school. Many of the same planning, response, command, and communications factors apply, and there is always the possibility children with special medical needs may be involved. The main difference with a bus incident off campus is that EMS will lack the instant presence of school staff and resources to assist and provide information because the driver may also be injured. National Highway Traffic Safety Administration accident data for the year 2006 includes 52,000 vehicle accidents involving buses with 299 fatalities of all types of crashes such as frontal or side impact and rollover.

Tracking students will be a major concern for EMS at school bus emergencies; even with detailed rosters of students on particular bus routes and a knowledgeable driver, there is usually some variability in the students actually onboard due to absences, students using an alternate bus due to after-school activities or sleepovers, and other special situations. Many school buses today are equipped with mobile radios, cell phones, or other two-way communications. After rescue and priority medical care have been managed, the priority will be reaching the school division's transportation director so that the school division's plan for parental notification can be initiated, and alternate transportation can be dispatched for any uninjured children.

The school system should address the following questions in its internal emergency plans, and each point should be discussed during preplanning meetings with EMS:

- Are buses and drivers included in the school or school division emergency plans, and are drivers involved in training and exercises?
- How would buses be mobilized and used during a major community emergency?
- Is there a mechanism for recalling buses/drivers during irregular transportation times?
- Is there a mutual aid agreement with neighboring school districts for mobilization of additional transportation resources?

Knowing the answers to these questions in advance can be valuable to EMS agencies when considering the usefulness and availability of school buses not only in MCIs at schools, but in large-incident and evacuation planning for the community. Bus availability and access can be incorporated into the medical transportation plans for school incidents as well as other community emergencies and evacuation scenarios.

An important part of planning for a school bus incident that should not be overlooked is scene safety at the bus crash site. Although this is considered by many as an operational incident consideration, it must be addressed with the same attention to detail as other aspects of school preplanning.

Incorporating the school bus incident into the overall school preplan permits the planners to address common issues such as the age of children and the incumbent difficulties with each age group, the possibility of parents showing up at the scene, and unique aspects of dealing with both of these issues in or near the roadway.

Because of these issues, preplanning must account for safety issues of multiple children both injured and uninjured, access and egress to and from the scene, staging of equipment, shutting down the roadway and coordination with law enforcement, and coordination with receiving medical facilities to deal with the patients, parents, and media.

## Preparing for School Emergencies

EMS planners must consider multiple variables when preplanning for incidents at schools, not the least of which is the capacity of occupants to self-rescue and follow instructions. The developmental stage of children and ratio of adult supervision will impact the number and type of EMS resources required at an emergency. Some level of emergency planning already exists in most schools and school systems due to accreditation and fire code requirements; EMS services can learn much from the American fire service's track record in preplanning and public education in schools.

The EMS preplanner must collect facts and make assumptions as a process to estimate the type of emergency incidents possible and EMS response required. Collaboration with other government resources and agencies will enhance the quality and detail level of the EMS preplan and result in EMS planners being more prepared during planning visits at schools. Existing planning tools such as school medical emergency response plans and emergency information forms are valuable for EMS responders; EMS agencies can serve as educators and community partners for schools by assisting school administrators where these documents do not already exist. Planners should utilize an organized process of data collection to assemble information for the preplan including facility, staff, and population details, as well as supporting documents and tools such as diagrams and site plans.

EMS preplans should integrate with and be complementary to existing fire department and other community emergency plans. Information obtained during the preplanning process may be used to establish specific dispatch alarm assignments and drive training for EMS agencies in many areas including mass-casualty operations and medical care for children with special needs.

Large incidents involving schools will most likely utilize unified command due to the size of the incident and multiple stakeholders involved including emergency responders, law enforcement, the school division, and local government. Communications provided by a JIC during and after a school emergency must be consistent and accurate due to the high level of community and media interest.

# Selected References

American Academy of Pediatrics, Committee on Pediatric Emergency Medicine, American College of Emergency Physicians and Pediatric Emergency Medicine Committee: Pediatric Mental Health Emergencies in the Emergency Medical Services System. *Pediatrics* 2006;118(4):1764–1767.

Carnevale, F, Alexander, E, et al.: Daily living with distress and enrichment: The moral experience of families with ventilator-assisted children at home. *Pediatrics* 2006;117(1):48–60.

Committee on Pediatric Emergency Medicine, Committee on Medical Liability, and the Task Force on Terrorism: The pediatrician and disaster preparedness. *Pediatrics* 2006;117(2):560–565.

Council on School Health: Disaster planning for schools. *Pediatrics* 2008;122(4):895–901.

Deickmann. MD and Ronald, A: *Pediatric Education for Prehospital Professionals.* 2nd ed. Sudbury, MA: Jones and Bartlett Publishers; 2006.

*Emergency Planning and Community Right to Know Act (EPCRA),* U.S. Code Title 42, Chapter 116; October, 1986.

Gagliardi, M, Neighbors, M, et al.: Emergencies in the school setting: Are public school teachers adequately trained to respond? *Prehosp Disaster Med* 1994;9:222–225.

Graham, J, Shirm, S, et al.: Mass casualty events at schools: A national preparedness survey. *Pediatrics* 2006; 117(1):e8–e15.

Hazinski, M, Markensen, D, et al. and the American Heart Association: Response to cardiac arrest and selected life-threatening medical emergencies: The medical emergency response plan for schools. *Circulation* 2004; 109(2):278–291.

Johnston, C and Redlener, I: Critical concepts for children in disasters identified by hands-on professionals: Summary of issues demanding solutions before the next one. *Pediatrics* 2006;117(5):S458–S460.

Kano, M, Ramirez, M, et al.: Are schools prepared for emergencies: A baseline assessment of emergency preparedness at school sites in three Los Angeles County school districts. *Educ Urban Soc* 2007;39:3399–3422.

Markenson, D, Reynolds, S, and Committee on Pediatric Emergency Medicine and Task Force on Terrorism: The pediatrician and disaster preparedness. *Pediatrics* 2006;117(2):340–362.

National Fire Protection Association: *Learn Not to Burn.* (A copyrighted curriculum for young children first implemented by the NFPA in 1978 and now in its third edition, part of the curriculum in more than 40,000 schools.) Quincy, MA: NFPA; 1978.

National Response Team Response Subcommittee Workgroup: *Joint Information Center Model: Collaborative Communications During Emergency Response.* Washington, D.C.: The National Response Team; 2000.

Occupational Health and Safety Administration. *Hazard Communication Standard.* 29 CFR 1910.1200.

Olness, K, Mandalakas, A, et al.: The children in disasters project: Addressing the special needs of children in man-made and natural disasters. *Pediatrics* 2008;121;S115.

Olympia, R, Wan, E, et al.: The preparedness of schools to respond to emergencies in children: A national survey of school nurses. *Pediatrics* 2005;116(6):e738–e745.

Reijneveld, S: Psychosocial implications of disaster on children and pediatric care. *Pediatrics* 2006;117(5): 1865–1866.

Smilde-van den Doel, D, Smit, C, et al.: School performance and social-emotional behavior of primary school children before and after a disaster. *Pediatrics* 2006;118(5):e1311–1320.

*The Drug Free Schools and Communities Act Amendments,* Public Law 101–226, 103 Stat. 1928; December 12, 1989.

United States Department of Transportation: *Traffic Safety Facts 2006: A Compilation of Motor Vehicle Crash Data from the Fatality Analysis Reporting System and the General Estimates System.* Washington, D.C.: DOT, National Center for Statistics and Analysis; 2006.

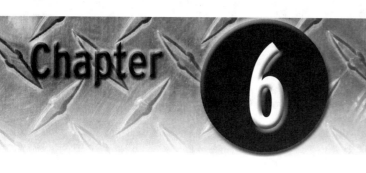

# Chapter 6

# Mass Gatherings

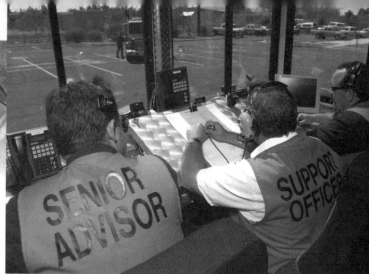

On January 20, 2009, hundreds of thousands of visitors thronged the Capitol for inauguration events in the January cold. The inauguration of the United States' first black president presented unique challenges for D.C. Fire and Emergency Medical Services (EMS). Long-experienced in handling the massive crowds that accompany political functions, Washington D.C. had implemented planning steps that included a state of emergency declaration by the mayor and federal assistance for the event, including activation of the Federal Emergency Management Agency's (FEMA's) ambulance contract to bring 100 additional ambulances to the city. D.C. Fire and EMS, their normal mutual aid partners from the National Capital and Baltimore area Council of Governments (COG), and ambulance strike teams from Maryland and Virginia provided another 100 ambulances.

Unique events provide learning opportunities for even the most experienced emergency care professionals. Between 4 am and 4 pm, EMS responded to 1,148 cases. While expecting massive crowds, city planners did not expect them to arrive so early. Though mutual aid resources were not scheduled to arrive until 6 am, fire officials reported visitors arriving as early as 1 am to claim viewing spots. As temperatures dropped into the teens that night and continued to fall throughout the morning, D.C. Fire and EMS used up a substantial portion of their planned resources in responding to a surge of EMS calls between 4 and 5 am. More than 400,000 visitors were in place on the Mall by 8:25 am; D.C. Fire and EMS responded to 262 EMS cases (including diabetic cases, cold-related illnesses, and falls) on the Mall between 4 and 10 am. At least one Metro station escalator failed under the weight of visitors, creating several calls for chest pain and breathing difficulty as visitors climbed from the underground station on the out-of-service escalator. Police eventually had to enforce maximum occupancy counts on Metro cars to avoid reported overwhelming crushing of passengers trying to fit into cars.

Though several public buildings remained open and planners had erected at least 40 warming tents in the inauguration areas, cold exposure cases occurred due to visitors' unwillingness to abandon their viewing spots. Four-hundred ninety people received care from providers in first aid tents and aid stations on the Mall; 31 of those patients were transported to hospitals.

## Introduction to Planning for Medical Care at Special Events

Response to injuries and illnesses at large special events can be challenging for EMS systems and event promoters because of crowd and traffic congestion (see **Figure 6-1**). Because of these challenges, a certain type of on-site medical care at mass gatherings has evolved into an expected standard in most communities. Whether provided by a volunteer rescue squad, municipal agency, or event management business, the design of an on-site medical care system for a special event is dependent on many variables. Planning for the delivery of special event medical care is a collaborative process that requires close coordination between venue owners, event promoters, medical providers, and surrounding jurisdictions and health systems.

Definitions for "special event" and "mass gathering" vary, and there is no consistently accepted attendance standard to qualify the event as a mass gathering. FEMA's Emergency Management Institute defines special event as "a nonroutine activity within a community that brings together a large number of people." Large mili-

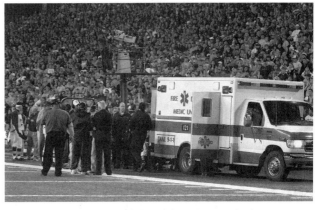

**Figure 6-1** Mass gatherings and special events present unique challenges to EMS.

tary air shows in the United States routinely exceed 250,000 spectators over a weekend. A half marathon with 500 participants may challenge a small EMS system if the heat index is extreme. Whether providing medical coverage for a state fair, concert, festival, or sporting event, an organized approach to planning can identify variables likely to influence the number of attendees who seek medical attention and help EMS planners identify strategies to provide effective special event medical coverage.

## Goal of Providing Event Medical Coverage

Prior to planning the specifics of medical coverage for a special event, EMS planners must first ask the question, "What is the medical coverage supposed to accomplish?" Event organizers request special event medical coverage for a variety of reasons. Limiting the event organizer's liability, reducing insurance premiums, improving the attendee experience, and complying with statutory, code, and zoning requirements are all potential reasons to provide medical coverage at large special events.

> **Special Event**
>
> A nonroutine activity within a community that brings together a large number of people.

The primary purpose of providing accessible medical care might be to:

- Provide convenient, on-site care for minor conditions to make it less likely that a customer will leave the event (and thus stop spending money at the event).
- Provide a community service to assist with restricted or lengthy egress due to crowd size, parking and traffic considerations, or remote location.
- Ensure a community's standard of EMS medical care remains consistent, even with the special circumstances of difficult access [eg, to provide "first shock" within 5 minutes of collapse or to provide an "advanced life support (ALS) on scene" response time of less than 9 minutes].
- Provide the minimum coverage necessary to satisfy requirements placed on the organizer by an insurance carrier or municipal code/regulation.
- Because it has always been done, and attendees expect it.

Only the event organizer and agency providing the medical coverage can determine the overall purpose or purposes of providing medical coverage. Early in the planning process, it is essential to determine the purpose of the coverage so that the EMS provider can establish planning and service goals, and event organizers can determine and outline a budget for providing the service.

# Negotiations for Event Medical Services

The National Association of EMS Physicians (NAEMSP) advocates a 15-step planning process for mass gathering medical care planning. One of the NAEMSP planning steps is "negotiating for event medical services." Many smaller community events, such as neighborhood festivals, parades, and 5-K runs, are often coordinated informally with a simple phone call to the EMS agency. In these cases, this is all that is required to secure a basic "EMS standby" at the event. This chapter intends to highlight planning considerations for all mass gathering possibilities, from a small community event to large events, such as an air show or celebration with hundreds of thousands of attendees. A more formal planning process should precede all but the smallest, most routine special events in order to ensure that human resources, financial, logistical, and liability issues are addressed among the event organizers and providers of EMS care.

Medical planners should consider the provision of EMS care at a special event a "business relationship" between the providers and the event organizer. A contractual relationship should exist between the EMS provider and event organizer. If a municipal EMS agency is providing coverage at a municipality-sponsored event at the direction of the city manager or county administrator, then a statutory arrangement already exists (since municipal code likely empowers the city manager to provide for public safety). If a nonprofit organization or for-profit business such as a promoter is the official organizer of an event, the EMS providers should insist on a formal contract with the organizers. The "contract" may range from a memorandum of agreement with a community nonprofit organization, to a formal contract with a promoter. EMS agency legal counsel and the medical director should be involved in determining the most appropriate type of contract.

According to *Mass Gathering Medical Care: The Medical Director's Checklist*, the following subjects should be negotiated and agreed upon in advance by the event organizers and EMS providers:

- Scope and responsibility for medical care, including medical direction and credentialing of EMS providers
- Financial responsibilities for EMS staff, equipment, and supplies
- Standard of coverage: number and type of EMS personnel
- Responsibility for liability insurance coverage for EMS personnel and the medical director
- Command, control, and reporting relationships among EMS personnel and event organizers

Compensation of the medical director and EMS providers should also be addressed during negotiations: Will an organizer have to reimburse a municipality for EMS provider overtime? Will any additional customer/patient fees result, that may be directly billed to the patient or insurance carrier, if an ambulance transport is necessary? If the EMS provider is a private service, rates and fees must be addressed, including any contractual penalties for the organizer and provider (eg, if the event runs longer than scheduled or if the EMS provider cannot meet staffing or response performance standards). If EMS providers are volunteers or will be assigned from normal daily EMS staffing, what "perks" can the organizer offer to ensure adequate volunteers and staff enthusiasm? Often promoters may offer free event tickets, event tee shirts, other souvenirs, or free or reduced-price meals to event staff. Any "perks" or incentives should be established and agreed upon in advance, to avoid ethical conflicts that could arise over a municipal employee receiving or asking for gifts. This also allows EMS personnel to be aware in advance of what "payment" they can expect.

# Liability and Risk Management

Event coordinators will most likely have to satisfy the venue operator that liability insurance is in place. It is also quite common for venue owners to require event coordinators to add the venue to the policy as an "additional insured" to general liability policies. A comprehensive risk management program that includes venue staff training and some level of on-site medical service can reduce insurance premiums. Comprehensive planning can maximize on-site response capabilities and reduce the consequences of accidents and illnesses that occur at the event. Many sporting leagues build requirements for event medical coverage into their venue and promoter certification requirements. The International Kickboxing Federation (IKF), for instance, requires a medical doctor and two paramedics equipped with resuscitation supplies and equipment to be on site for all IKF-sanctioned events.

Some states specifically provide civil immunity for organizers and advertisers of community events and functions. It is generally recognized, however, that most "good Samaritan" legislation does not completely protect EMS providers and physicians from medical liability, particularly when the providers are paid or when other contractual relationships exist. Payment of volunteers and criminal background checks of event organizers and volunteers are other issues that should be considered carefully. The EMS agency's staff legal counsel and insurance carrier should be consulted for specific guidance. Physicians should consult their liability and malpractice insurance carrier to determine if their general malpractice policy covers their work as a special event provider or medical director, or if additional insurance riders are needed.

Many local, state, or federal governments are "self-insured;" events coordinated by government agencies likely fall under the government's general liability. Self-insured government organizations usually employ a formal, organized risk assessment and management strategy. Whether an agency falls under a self-insured government or not, an organized program of risk assessment and risk management can reduce accidents and injuries and reduce the organization's exposure to liability. An injury surveillance system that would track sporting event spectator injuries and deaths, for example, would allow spectators to make intelligent decisions about the level of risk they are willing to accept and assist the venue industry, promoters, and insurance providers to quantify and address the risk.

# Level of Care

Many variables, not the least of which is financial, must be considered to establish what the required level of care will be at a given event. EMS planners should use the negotiated medical coverage contract to develop a plan for the event. The community's existing standard may serve as a guide for large events sponsored by a municipality. In planning for a large outdoor festival covering several acres of a city park, for example, EMS might plan for the area to be patrolled by ALS providers, if that is the standard that is provided elsewhere in the community. This may be necessary, particularly if access to the event could be delayed for providers responding in from outside the event. At a large event that extends over more than a single day, it may be advantageous to utilize an on-site physician, particularly if a high number of patients is anticipated. Other than providing a physician level of care, the on-site physician can also provide on-site medical direction for EMS personnel and be responsible for treat-and-release and "no transport" determinations. One California study demonstrated that on-site physicians may reduce hospital transports from special events up by as much as 89 percent.

For general planning purposes, the NAEMSP recommends an emergency medical technician (EMT) equipped with defibrillation capability as the minimum acceptable level of care at mass gatherings. Furthermore, for planning for the deployment of personnel at events, the NAEMSP advocates that an EMT with defibrillator be able to access a patient who collapses within 5 minutes.

A tiered deployment plan may be beneficial and allow EMS to conserve more highly skilled resources. Physicians and ALS providers may provide primary care at the base of operations, while patrol and inter-event transportation is provided by both basic life support (BLS) and ALS teams. If multiple fixed locations are staffed, a physician may staff the base of operations and provide medical direction and oversight, while paramedics and nurses staff remote sites. Physicians working at large special events have been observed to reduce the demand on local hospitals and to improve patient care documentation. When an event covers a very large area, such as a 10-K, half marathon, or other long-distance course, it is reasonable to concentrate physician-level care at fixed locations (such as start and finish lines), provide ALS-staffed intravenue and extravenue transportation, and provide BLS with defibrillation capabilities at points along the route.

Protocols must be addressed by medical direction and EMS planners, particularly if a large event will be staffed by EMS providers from multiple agencies or jurisdictions. Ideally, the community's existing protocols should be used to avoid provider confusion. EMS staff from outside the normal jurisdiction should be provided event protocol information and training in advance. When the purpose of special event medical coverage is to keep the attendees engaged and present at the event, or if access and egress is extremely limited by crowds and traffic, it may be advantageous to plan for special event protocols. For instance, EMS providers in many jurisdictions do not normally dispense over-the-counter remedies such as analgesics and antacids, but this service may be desirable at a large event. Treat and release protocols may be utilized at events involving high heat and humidity in order to provide oral or intravenous rehydration prior to determining if a patient must be transported to a hospital. Intuitively, these types of special event protocols seem like a good idea and may reduce the demand on transport resources and reduce hospital visits. However, providers must be familiar with the protocols, and close supervision and medical direction are essential for their success.

## Planning Documents, Forms, and Record Keeping

When preplanning for mass gatherings, it is important for EMS to implement effective documentation of all aspects of plan development.

### Incident Action Plan

A major principle of the incident command system is that every incident should have an incident action plan (IAP). Fire and EMS responses utilize agency standard operating procedures and practices as the IAP. For instance, an agency's standard IAP for a single motor-vehicle collision will likely include the following objectives:

- Control traffic and protect the scene.
- Stabilize the vehicle.
- Access the patient.
- Extricate the patient.
- Provide emergency care and transport.
- Return the scene to normal conditions.

A written IAP is generally not prepared for routine emergencies addressed by common response plans and procedures. An event that requires multi-agency work and planning and that is outside of the norm of day-to-day responses should have a written IAP to address objectives, specific responsibilities, and resources required to manage the event. The IAP must be divided into operational periods for long or multi-day events. An IAP should contain strategic goals, tactical objectives, and needed support.

Based on the size and complexity of the event, the IAP may also contain the following:

- *Event timeline.* Special security situations, such as a presidential visit, and events with multiple activities over several days, such as a community festival involving a 5-K run, musical performances, and other activities, should have a timeline that indicates the times and sequence of events and their locations included in the IAP.
- *Medical action plan.* The NAEMSP advocates a detailed medical action plan for all events that require on-site medical resources. The medical action plan serves as an operational component or annex to the IAP. Local government, through zoning and permitting officials, may also require event organizers to submit a written medical plan as part of the application process for obtaining a special-use permit.
- *Traffic management plan.* High-attendance events that could impact normal traffic flow and parking availability should include a traffic management plan.
- *Security plan.* Based on the type of event and need for security resources, a security plan should be developed.

Command meetings to develop the IAP should include representatives from the various agencies and organizations that are stakeholders in the event. Even a small, community special event operating with a single incident command versus a unified command will have multiple stakeholders and organizers including the local government, venue management, police and security, fire and EMS, and recreation or festival planners. According to FEMA, during the initial command meeting, each participating agency and jurisdiction should:

- State its organizational objectives; these objectives should be edited and combined into a collective, single set of incident objectives for the IAP.
- Present jurisdictional and agency limitations, restrictions, and concerns.
- Establish and agree on accepted priorities.
- Adopt a general, overall strategy or strategies to accomplish the incident objectives.
- Agree on the basic structure of the command organization.
- Agree on the best qualified operations section chief.
- Agree on general staff personnel designations as well as planning, logistical, and financing arrangements and procedures.
- Agree on the resource ordering process to be followed.
- Agree on cost-sharing procedures.
- Agree on public information policies to be followed.
- Designate a single official to act as the command spokesperson.

Using a cooperative planning process that adheres to the principles of incident command will result in a cohesive IAP that addresses multi-agency concerns and priorities while specifying operational tactics and resource assignments for the cooperative effort.

## Medical Action Plan

The medical action plan is a specific component of the IAP that addresses all aspects of medical coverage to be delivered on site and may be an important reference of the contract between medical providers and

### Incident Action Plan

A written or oral plan that covers strategic goals, tactical objectives, and support resources required for an incident or event. Depending on the length of the event, more than one IAP may be needed, or it may be necessary to divide the IAP into operational periods.

### General Staff

Under the incident command system, the incident commander's general staff are managers that direct operations, planning, finance/administration, and logistics sections. These general staff directors carry the title of section chief.

the event organizers. The medical action plan should address human resources, liability and insurance, finance, and all other aspects of on-site medical care. Ideally, the medical action plan should be finalized and approved by the EMS coordinator and medical director at least 30 days prior to the event. Copies of the medical action plan should be provided to all government agencies that are involved with the event and any adjoining EMS agencies or other resources that are referenced in the plan. All medical supervisors and team leaders should be familiarized with the plan prior to the event. Medical technicians and individual providers can be briefed on their specific assignments, objectives, and "all hands" information, such as communications at operational briefings at the start of each shift.

## Record Keeping

Forms should be provided for the medical branch director to track personnel and equipment. The EMS planner, event medical director, and event organizers must determine how patient contacts will be documented. If the medical standby is being provided by a municipal EMS agency, using the agency's standard paper or electronic prehospital patient care report will result in less confusion for medical providers. Supplemental paper or forms should be available for physicians, nurse practitioners, and other advanced providers to document patient assessment and treatment at fixed points of care. Planners must also consider how to document minor conditions and walk-up requests that do not necessarily warrant a complete physical examination or completion of a standard call report. Many agencies utilize a log to check patients in and out of treatment areas and document minor care such as dispensing over-the-counter medications and providing minor wound care.

When planning the methods for documenting patient care, planners and medical directors must contemplate what data will need to be extracted for quality management purposes and future event planning. Whether paper or electronic, patient care record-keeping systems should be designed to track key criteria of interest to the agency and medical director, such as the total number of patient contacts, patient chief complaints, patients seen by a physician, patients transported off site for care, patients treated and released, patients who refused care against medical advice, types of interventions performed, and medications dispensed.

The format and form of "refusal of care" documents should be agreed upon in advance. Professional athletic circuit promoters often have developed their own waiver or patient refusal form. Most EMS agencies utilize refusal forms whenever patients decline care or transportation. Legal counsel should be consulted to ensure that the refusal form used is adequate to protect EMS providers and medical direction. The refusal form chosen should be provided and explained to all medical providers.

## Staff Health and Safety

The safety of medical branch staff should be specifically addressed in the IAP. An accountability system should be utilized, and periodic roll calls performed to verify the status and presence of medical staff members. Staff members should receive advance communication regarding specific event characteristics and their assignments so that appropriate uniforms, clothing, and shoes can be selected. If staff are to be stationed outdoors, foul weather gear should be provided if necessary. For medical staff members using bicycles, recreational trail vehicle-style carts, and other special response equipment, the appropriate personal protective equipment should be issued. Medical providers should be reminded to monitor their own health and that of their teammates, and to be attentive to hydration (see **Figure 6-2**). Rest periods and meal breaks should be provided. EMS planners should consider creating a checklist or staff roster specifically to track breaks and accountability checks to ensure that all staff members receive rest and meals.

## Planning Resources

Many resources exist to assist event and medical planners in the various specific disciplines involved in planning a large event. The US Department of Transportation publishes the *Managing Travel for Planned Special Events* handbook, which is available on the Federal Highway Administration publications web site. FEMA's Emergency Management Institute offers the free, online course, *Special Events Contingency Planning for Public Safety Agencies* (available at www.training.fema.gov/EMIWeb/IS/IS15a.asp). The Pennsylvania Emergency Management Agency has published the *Special Event Emergency Action Plan Guide*. The NAEMSP Standards and Clinical Practice Committee publishes the *Mass Gathering Medical Care: The Medical Director's Checklist*. The checklist is actually a small book with comprehensive recommendations categorized as either essential or desirable. The checklist is available from the NAEMSP.

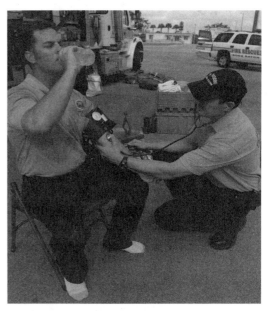

**Figure 6-2** The safety of the involved emergency responders should be specifically addressed in an IAP.

# Event Reconnaissance

A careful review and reconnaissance of all aspects of the event should be undertaken to aid planning activities. The characteristics of the expected event participants and attendees and the physical characteristics of the venue are two critical components of a thorough reconnaissance.

## Prediction of Patient Presentation

Published medical literature contains many reports of attempts to accurately predict patient presentation rates and chief complaints, none of which have been validated. The most accurate method known to predict patient presentation rates is to draw on past experience with a specific event or venue. Even this method is subject to variabilities in crowd, weather, and other factors. In the absence of event-specific historical data, planners must make educated guesses based on assumptions about the variables associated with the event. It might be assumed, for instance, that a "senior olympics" event will have a higher patient presentation rate because of biomedical reasons, namely the age and physical condition of the participants.

Andrew Milsten analyzed 4 years of attendance data at National Football League games held at Baltimore Ravens stadium and found 1,887 patients presented at first aid stations out of a total of more than 2.5 million attendees. This is an average rate of one out of every 1,395 guests presenting to a first aid station. Approximately one of every 11 patients seen in first aid stations was transported offsite for medical attention.

Risk and hazard assessment should be performed to quantify event variables in advance, particularly for outdoor events. An effort should be made to identify hazards that might impact attendees. Weather reports and predictions should be monitored up to and during the event, and forecasted weather extremes should be addressed in the IAP. The Pennsylvania Emergency Management Association's *Special Event Emergency Action Plan Guide* provides an excellent

## Crowd Management

Effectively organizing the movement of crowds. Understanding basic crowd behavior assists event managers in formulating effective plans, which should be adjusted to meet the needs of the event and the specific crowd.

## Crowd Control

Steps taken once a crowd (or sections of it) begins to behave in a dangerous or unruly manner.

checklist matrix for predicting the potential of risk based on specific hazards. Once the level of risk of a specific hazard is established, planners can determine whether it needs to be addressed as a contingency in the IAP.

## Crowd

While crowd management and crowd control are not typically a responsibility of the EMS or medical section of a special event, it should be addressed in the IAP, and medical planners must have a basic knowledge of how the crowd "personality" may influence event planning. A crowd can take on a personality much different from the majority of individuals in the crowd. Event participants may assume one of the following roles in a crowd:

- *Observers.* Follow the actions of a crowd, but rarely take part
- *Cheerleaders.* May not directly participate in the crowd's actions, but provide verbal support and encouragement to the crowd's leaders
- *Active core.* Carries out the actions of the crowd

The influence of alcohol and drugs may significantly impact the behavior of a crowd and the tendency toward accidents or medical emergencies. Crowd size and personalities may increase the probability of a dangerous occurrence, increase the potential number of victims, make communications and response slower and more difficult, and tend to diffuse responsibility (each section thinks another section is responsible for carrying out a task).

### Physical Characteristics of Venue

While specific considerations for point-of-care locations are offered later in the chapter, there are many other venue features and characteristics that should be evaluated during reconnaissance. Overall size and layout of the venue or event location will influence the location of fixed-care sites and personnel deployment. Physical barriers (such as crowd fencing at an air show, security gates and turnstiles at concert venues, and concrete barriers and fencing around a race track) will influence response capabilities and affect response times. Restroom facilities, food concession location, and access to potable and non-potable water may influence crowd patterns. Temporary power distribution systems and the presence of gas cylinders for cooking and grilling at outdoor festivals create special hazards. For outdoor events, available shelter opportunities should be identified in the event of a severe storm. Access to and egress from the event as well as a staging location for ambulances and other transport resources should be scouted in advance and incorporated into the medical action plan.

Area hospitals and their specific capabilities [eg, trauma center, pediatric specialty, stroke center, ST-segment elevation myocardial infarction (STEMI) center] should be identified in advance. If resources from outside the jurisdiction will be utilized for patient transportation, packets should be prepared with contact information and driving directions to area hospitals.

In *Mass Gathering Medical Care: The Medical Director's Checklist*, David Jaslow, Arthur Yancey, and Andrew Milsten also advocate for the evaluation of the following during event reconnaissance:

- Potential for warm ambient temperature and heat-related illnesses
- Potential for cold ambient temperature and cold-related illnesses
- Precipitation, threat of storms, and unexpected changes in temperature
- Ground conditions: terrain, wet and slippery versus dry

- Availability of food and water for attendees
- Law enforcement and venue security presence
- Presence of dignitaries, VIPs
- Threats against the event and other security concerns
- Likelihood of event- or location-specific disaster (tornado-prone areas, aircraft or race car crash)

Sporting events often offer event-specific hazards for participants that must be planned for and addressed in the plan. "Extreme" sports, long distance runs, obstacle/challenge courses, boxing, wrestling, and similar activities may drive the need for on-site EMS even when the crowd is not expected to be exceptionally large.

# EMS Delivery: Point of Care

The type of venue, type and length of the event, as well as predictions of the number and types of potential patient contacts will drive decision making concerning exactly where medical services will be delivered. Available resources (number of potential staff and diagnostic equipment) will also figure in to the point-of-care design, as will the level of care to be delivered.

## Fixed Location

At all but the shortest events, medical providers will need a place to stage equipment, store personal items, and perform command and record-keeping tasks. A fixed location, either permanent or portable, provides a base from which to operate as well as a walk-up location and treatment area for patients.

## Permanent Fixed Location

Concert halls and arenas, fairgrounds, parks, and other public facilities often have designated rooms within the facility for first-aid, particularly if designed within the past decade. These facilities range from a small room in a civic center, to first-aid rooms on multiple levels of larger arenas, to fully equipped, free-standing urgent care centers in the infield of modern automobile race tracks. Although certain types are recommended for the facility by architects and public safety officials, the providers of medical care at public, multi-use facilities may vary due to the types of events. The municipal owner of an arena may require a concert promoter to provide EMS coverage for a concert, while the municipality itself provides EMS coverage for a high school sports tournament at the same facility. Due to multiple providers utilizing the location, it may be furnished, but may not be supplied and equipped.

Facility reconnaissance in advance will reveal important planning considerations specific to the event and dictate the type of advance logistics support that will be necessary. Fixed structures offer many advantages over portable structures, but there are still important planning considerations to identify during reconnaissance:

- *Personal storage.* Is there a secure location for providers to store personal items while on duty? Providers should be advised in advance to minimize the amount of personal items such as purses, jackets, etc, if secure storage is not available.
- *Medication storage.* Is there regulation-compliant, locking storage for controlled substances? Lack of adequate controlled substance storage may limit the types of medications the provider can have available.
- Is the location stocked with necessary equipment and supplies?

## Portable Fixed Location

Organizations that routinely provide special event EMS coverage often invest in portable facilities and structures that can serve as a treatment facility and base of operations at locations without permanent areas for medical care. Easily deployed, pop-up style shelters are often used during running events as well as outdoor fairs and festivals. Larger tents with sides, doors, and even room dividers are effective as a temporary base of operations for larger events. Combinations of larger and smaller shelters may be used at very large, more geographically dispersed events.

Trailers equipped with awnings, generators, and climate control can serve as treatment locations and operations bases, as well as storage areas for special event supplies and equipment. Larger agencies and health systems have utilized custom-built recreational vehicles and semi-trailers as mobile clinics.

When using a portable fixed location, specific reconnaissance items to assess include:

- *Surface type and drainage.* Will the medical shelter be operating on top of a mud pit if it rains?
- *Proximity to electricity.* If utilizing base station radios, vital sign monitors, and other electronic equipment or lighting, is the location within close proximity to a power source? Is the pathway for power cords protected to prevent damage to the cords and trip hazards?
- *Generator location.* If power is to be provided by a generator, is there a location suitable for generator placement that will reduce the level of generator noise and exhaust fumes in the treatment area and allow for safe refueling operations?
- *Safety and identification.* Does the selected location allow for guidelines and tent stakes to be installed without intruding into egress and crowd movement pathways? What is the method of marking or flagging guidelines, wires, and tent stakes to prevent a guest from walking into or tripping over the equipment? What method can be used to identify the portable facility as an EMS station?
- *Sanitary facilities.* The location of the closest restrooms and running water should be identified for providers. The method and location of garbage disposal should also be identified in advance with the event coordinators.
- *Patient privacy.* Can the structure be partitioned to allow for some privacy while examining a patient or can an ambulance be staged nearby to provide privacy?

No matter which point of service is utilized, planners must address supplies and equipment needed for the level of care being provided. Particular attention should be paid to supplies and equipment cached for special events or stored at permanent, fixed facilities. Biomedical devices and durable medical equipment such as stretchers must be maintained in accordance with Food and Drug Administration (FDA) requirements and manufacturer recommendations. Expiration dates, medications, and consumable medical supplies must be monitored.

## Intravenue Transportation

Once the venue has been examined, planners should assess possible mechanisms of moving nonambulatory patients to fixed treatment areas. As with normal EMS calls, patients will present with a wide range of mobility assistance needs. There should be a method to move patients who are completely nonambulatory because of a medical emergency, as well as patients who may be too weak or elderly to walk a long distance. Inside concert arenas, civic centers, and convention halls with wide passageways and elevators, wheeled stretchers and wheelchairs may be sufficient. At larger venues and outdoor events, specially constructed golf carts and recreational trail vehicles (RTVs) equipped with litters and EMS equipment are often used to navigate crowded areas where use of an ambulance is impractical. Resource requests for these vehicles and equipment should be made in advance as part of the event planning process. While golf carts and RTVs are widely used for recreational and utility purposes, these are specialized vehicles; operator safety and training should be emphasized, and standard operating procedures detailing their use should be implemented.

### Extravenue Transportation

Ambulance and nonurgent transportation for off-site medical care should be addressed in the plan. Planners should avoid using ambulance crews for other staff positions in the medical branch if their ambulances are part of the transportation plan; pulling that crew for a transport would leave their positions uncovered. Past experience, availability of ambulance resources, and ease of access to the venue all contribute to determination of the number of ambulances needed to be on site in staging. Any standby fees and transport billing arrangements should be made as part of the event negotiations process. Event planners should enter into contracts with private ambulance services and mutual aid agreements with municipal ambulance services to ensure liability, employee injury, workers' compensation, and financial reimbursement issues are addressed and agreed upon by all parties.

On the basis of the type and number of patient contacts expected and availability of ambulances, EMS planners should consider transportation options for patients with subacute conditions who do not require transport on a stretcher. Patients may be incapacitated to the point that assistance is required and they should not drive, but they may not require the services of an entire EMS crew and stretcher transportation. Sedans or minivans with a driver may be used for this purpose; some jurisdictions have utilized parks and recreation department staff, vehicles, and taxicab vouchers for this purpose. State EMS regulations should be consulted to verify under what conditions patient transport can be conducted in this manner and to determine whether licensing of nonambulance-type vehicles is required. If not on site, planners should have a resource list of companies that can provide wheelchair transportation.

## Accessing EMS

A plan must be developed to educate event attendees and event staff on how to access EMS at the event. On the basis of the venue characteristics, there may need to be many mechanisms available to access EMS. Other than a method for visitors to access EMS, the key to delivering an effective response is a dedicated calltaker and dispatcher onsite in the medical branch or shared with event security. The following lists different ways to let event attendees know how to access EMS.

- *Public address announcements.* Announcers should be provided scripts or information cards and periodically announce the location of first aid stations.
- *Event security.* The visitor's first contact when emergency services are needed may be a security guard or police officer assigned to the event. There must be a communications link between security and EMS to relay requests for service.
- *Event staff.* The paid and volunteer staffs at large community and sporting events often utilize radio or cell phone push-to-talk communications for event coordination purposes. Event staff should receive basic education on the medical action plan and location of first aid stations. There must be a communications link between event staff and EMS to relay requests for service.

The advance of convenient and economical technology provides a special complication for emergency services at large special events: When attendees cannot easily locate a security or event staff member, they often call 9-1-1 utilizing their cell phone. The jurisdiction's emergency communications center (ECC) should be involved in the event planning, and receive notification whenever an organic medical or EMS capability will be operating at a special event. Ideally, the ECC can designate a tactical channel for exclusive use by the event medical staff, and designate a tactical channel for command communications and for the relay of requests for service from the ECC to the event medical branch. Otherwise, a 9-1-1 call may result in the ECC sending predesignated response resources to the venue without onsite EMS being aware of the emergency.

Another consideration for cell phone 9-1-1 calls is the proximity of the venue to jurisdictional boundaries. Cell phone 9-1-1 calls may even reach an ECC outside the venue's jurisdiction based on cell tower usage volume, atmospheric conditions, and other variables. Cell towers located adjacent to US highways and interstates are often programmed to relay 9-1-1 calls to a state police dispatcher versus the local jurisdiction. All of these factors must be considered, and notification and communications planning with multiple jurisdictions and ECCs may be necessary.

# Contingency Planning

EMS must conduct efficient contingency planning prior to a mass-gathering incident. This involves close consideration of special security situations and response needs for mass-casualty incidents (MCIs).

## Special Security Situations

Event organizers should have their security specialists liaison with local law enforcement for general notification and planning purposes, particularly traffic and crowd management. This liaison provides a link to law enforcement for important notifications about security threats such as protesters and threats of terrorism. Law enforcement and security liaisons may have intelligence that dictates extra precautions be taken for certain events, such as having nerve agent antidotes present on scene for use by medical providers.

Some events by their very nature are considered special security events due to the presence of politicians or VIPs. The director of the Department of Homeland Security has the authority to declare an event to be national special security event (NSSE) if the social, political, religious, or other cultural significance of the event increases the likelihood that it will be targeted by terrorists or other criminal activity. Visits by politicians and other dignitaries may also result in special security requirements. EMS planners will note that US Secret Service personnel (responsible for NSSEs and protection details for national political figures) are much more interested and involved in medical planning than their local law enforcement counterparts. The planning process is the same, but with additional interaction and collaboration with security planners. Additionally, certain portions or the entirety of the IAP, medical action plan, and other event information may be designated as "public safety sensitive" with distribution restricted to the relevant public safety personnel.

## MCI Planning

Large special events have the potential to turn into MCI events. As part of the risk management and event reconnaissance process of developing the medical action plan, EMS planners should evaluate the possibility of an MCI developing at the event. Certain activities have more risk than others: The nature of the event, security intelligence, and other factors must be analyzed to make a determination of what, if any, actions should be taken to address the potential of an MCI as a contingency.

At the very least, the medical branch staff should receive assignments of what their roles will be, should an MCI develop. The medical branch director essentially assigns members to positions in two parallel organizational structures at the beginning of their shift. For example, the nurse at first aid station 1 may be assigned the primary role of "leader" or "attendant in charge" at first aid station 1, and in the event of an MCI, his or her role might shift to "treatment group leader." The EMT-B working with the nurse at first aid station 1 has the primary duty as a medical provider in the first aid station, but in the event of an MCI, his or her assignment changes to "red treatment team leader."

Providers and staff should also receive instructions on where to report, should an MCI develop, and receive assignments for who is to retrieve and move equipment and supply caches.

Identification vests and checklists should be provided to personnel for their dual-role MCI assignment at the start of their shift or be cached for quick distribution when providers report to the designated rally point/staging area for their MCI assignment.

It may also be prudent at very large events to prestage MCI resources closer to the event so that response is not hampered by crowds and traffic. MCI supply vehicles and trailers may be positioned in close proximity to the event. The medical branch direction should plan for personnel assignments to retrieve and deploy these resources if needed for an MCI.

## Preplanning Considerations for Special Events

Planning for special event medical care is a collaborative process involving event promoters, venue owners, medical providers, local government, and other service providers with roles to play in successful event organization. Planners should first establish what the purpose and expectations of event medical coverage are and then establish service delivery goals and initiate the planning process. A businesslike relationship should be established between event organizers and EMS planners, with formal agreements and plans that address medical direction, finance, liability, as well as roles and responsibilities. A formal medical action plan should be researched, formulated, approved, and published at least 30 days in advance of the event. With the addition of a section on EMS provider health and safety, the 15-item NAEMSP medical action plan format is ideal for this purpose. The medical action plan should tie into the event's IAP, and medical staff accountability and supervisory relationships should be accounted for in the event's incident command organization. Hazard and risk assessment principles should be used to identify contingencies such as severe weather, security risks, and potential for MCIs.

## Selected References

Abbott, JL and Geddie, MW: Event and venue management: Minimizing liability through effective crowd management techniques. *Event Management* 2001;6:259–270.

Arbon, P: The development of conceptual models for mass-gathering health. *Prehosp Disaster Med* 2004;19(3):208–212.

Arbon, P, Bridgewater, F, et al.: Mass gathering medicine: A predictive model for patient presentation and transport rates. *Prehosp Disaster Med* 2001;16(3):109–116.

Calabro, J, Krohmer, J, et al.: *Provision of Emergency Medical Care for Crowds.* American College of Emergency Physicians EMS Committee; 1995–1996.

Emergency Management Institute: Federal emergency management administration course IS-15.a, in *Special Events Contingency Planning for Public Safety Agencies.* http://training.fema.gov/EMIWeb/IS/IS15a.asp. Accessed December 1, 2009.

Feldman, M, Lukins, J, et al.: Half-a-million strong: The emergency medical services response to a single-day, mass-gathering event. *Prehosp Disaster Med* 2004;19(4):287–296.

Flabouris, A, Nocera, A, et al.: Efficacy of critical incident monitoring for evaluating disaster medical readiness and response during the Sydney 2000 olympic games. *Prehosp Disaster Med* 2004;19(2):164–168.

Goss, KC: Emergency management & special events: Challenges, support, best practices. *DomPrep Journal* 2004;5:12–13.

Grange, JT: Planning for large events. *Current Sports Medicine Reports.* 2002;1(3):156–161.

Grange, JT, Baumann, GW, et al.: On-site physicians reduce ambulance transports at mass gatherings. *Prehosp Emerg Care* 2003;7:322–326.

International Kickboxing Federation: *Event Medical Staff Information and Requirements.* http://www.ikfkickboxing.com/Physicians.htm. Accessed December 1, 2009.

Jasolow, D, Yancey II, A, et al.: *Mass Gathering Medical Care: The Medical Director's Checklist.* Lenexa, KS: National Association of EMS Physicians; 2000.

Jolly, BT and Martinez, R: Heart stopping action: Whether it's a sporting event or rock concert, medical emergencies can spoil the fun and create liability unless management plans ahead. *Security Management*; April, 2004.

Leonard, RB, Winslow, JE, et al.: Planning medical care for high-risk mass gatherings. *Internet Journal of Rescue and Disaster Medicine* 2007;6(1).

Lukins, JL, Feldman MJ, et al.: A paramedic-staffed rehydration unit at a mass gathering. *Prehosp Emerg Care* 2004;8(4):411–416.

Ma, OJ, Millward, L, et al.: EMS medical coverage at PGA tour events. *Prehosp Emerg Care* 2002;6(1):11–14.

Milsten, AM: *From Start to Finish: Physician Usefulness at Mass Gathering Event.* American College of Emergency Physicians; 2009. http://www.acep.org/ACEPmembership.

Milsten, A, Maguire, B, et al.: Mass-gathering medical care: A review of the literature. *Prehosp Disaster Med* 2002;17(3):151–162.

Milsten, A, Seaman, K, et al.: Variables influencing medical usage rates, injury patterns, and levels of care for mass gatherings. *Prehosp Disaster Med* 2003;18(4):334–346.

Morimura, N, Katsumi, A, et al.: Analysis of patient load data from the 2002 FIFA World Cup Korea/Japan. *Prehosp Disaster Med* 2004;19(3):278–284.

Pennsylvania Emergency Management Agency: *Special Event Emergency Action Plan Guide.* Harrisburg, PA: Pennsylvania Emergency Management Agency. http://www.portal.state.pa.us. Accessed December 1, 2009.

Salhanick, S, Shehan, W, et al.: Use and analysis of field triage criteria for mass gathering. *Prehosp Disaster Med* 2003;18(4):347–352.

Sanderson, P: Liability involving special events, in *New Hampshire Town & City.* Concord, NH: New Hampshire Local Government Center; May, 2009.

Schulte, D and Meade, DM: The Papal chase. The Pope's visit: A 'mass' gathering. *Emerg Med Services* 1993;22(1):46–49, 65–75, 79.

Snowden, L and Kyle, L S: Crowds, cold challenge D.C. responders at inauguration. *EMSResponder.com*; January 20, 2009.

Snowden, L and Kyle, LS: Inaugural response: An inside look. *EMSResponder.com*; January 18, 2009.

Thierbach, A, Wolcke, B, et al.: Medical support for children's mass gatherings. *Prehosp Disaster Med* 2003;18(1):14–19.

United States Department of Homeland Security: Incident management: Alerting hospitals in close proximity to a mass casualty incident. *Lessons Learned Information Sharing.* https://www.llis.dhs.gov/index.do.

United States Department of Transportation: Managing travel for planned special events, in *Publication No: FHWA-NHI-03-120.* Washington, D.C.: DOT; 2003. http://www.ops.fhwa.dot.gov/publications. Accessed December 1, 2009.

Winslow, JE and Goldstein, AO: Spectator risks at sporting events. *The Internet Journal of Law, Healthcare and Ethics* 2007;4:2.

# Chapter 7

# Planning for Mass Medical Transportation

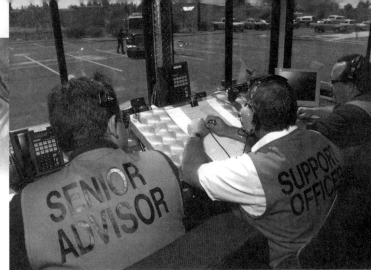

## Case Study

In the days prior to August 29, 2005, with Hurricane Katrina approaching the New Orleans metropolitan area, a decision had to be made: Evacuate the area or ride out the storm. Due to the ferocity of the coming hurricane, many assisted living facilities and nursing homes made the decision to evacuate their residents to higher ground. Out of 60 nursing homes in the New Orleans area, 21 evacuated their residents in advance of the hurricane. In most cases, this involved transporting bedridden patients over 100 miles to a safer area.

To accomplish such a large-scale evacuation, a large number of ambulances were required, and strained local emergency medical services (EMS) resources, which were already strained due to the evacuation orders in effect for their own personnel and their families. Transporting these often fragile patients over such a long distance, however, is not without potential complications. In fact, the first hurricane-related deaths occurred the day before Hurricane Katrina struck when three residents died while being evacuated to Baton Rouge. In contrast, over half the nursing homes in New Orleans decided against early evacuation. It was widely felt that many residents would not survive evacuation, and so no preparations were made. Eventually, this would prove to be a deadly mistake for several facilities, and at the top of the list was St. Rita's Nursing Home outside of Chalmette, LA.

In the days prior to the hurricane, when other facilities were evacuating their residents to safety, the operators of St. Rita's made the decision to shelter-in-place. After Hurricane Katrina made landfall, it was apparent that this was the wrong decision, and led to the drowning deaths of 35 residents.

Were these deaths the fault of EMS for not mandating the move to safety? Ultimately, in the case of St. Rita's, the finger was pointed at the facility operators for failing to evacuate their residents. Without preplanning and preparation for hurricane evacuations, instances such as this could easily have been blamed on EMS.

With the large numbers of bedridden patients requiring evacuation in the face of a hurricane, EMS agencies must be prepared, through preplanning, to have an adequate number of vehicles ready and available for safe evacuations.

## Transportation Considerations During Emergency Response

A wide variety of emergency situations may result in an order or recommendation for a community's evacuation. Many facilities and some private homes will be faced with the movement of nonambulatory persons. While careful advance planning by health care facilities will result in smooth patient movement for some, EMS planners must assume that some facilities and individuals in the community will require assistance (see **Figure 7-1**).

State laws on exactly who may order a mandatory evacuation vary. In some states, the chief local elected official may order mandatory evacuations. In others, local officials may only recommend evacuation, while the authority to order mandatory evacuation is reserved for the governor. The official with the authority to order or recommend evacuation relies on information and recommendations from emergency management officials.

EMS may be tasked with providing and/or coordinating the following, in addition to normal 9-1-1 service:

- Transportation from private residences and evacuating licensed care facilities to medical needs shelters
- Transportation from medical needs shelters to hospitals
- Transportation for nonambulatory patients from personal residences and evacuating licensed care facilities to licensed care facilities outside the disaster area
- Transportation from evacuating hospitals to other hospitals outside the disaster area
- Transportation to or from a national disaster medical system (NDMS) debarkation point or patient reception area (PRA)

EMS planners must address both "notice" and "no-notice" events. In a "notice" event, agencies may have a period of hours or days to prepare by obtaining additional supplies, scheduling staff, relocating resources, and implementing contracts. An example of a "notice" event is a hurricane, with a forecasted track and advance public announcements and evacuation recommendations. A "no-notice" event such as an earthquake or large hazardous materials or transportation accident provides the same challenges as a "notice" event, but with little or no advance warning.

As with other EMS planning activities, planning for large-scale transportation should start with an estimation to characterize the threat based on known facts and some assumptions.

## Evacuation Planning Assumptions

Emergency management officials must make some assumptions in order to plan. **Table 7-1** outlines local government responsibilities during evacuation. Planning assumptions used by emergency managers may be helpful to EMS planners for estimating the resources that will be required to assist in the evacuation on nonambulatory residents:

- Most people at risk will evacuate when local officials recommend they do so. Generally, 75% to 80% of those at risk will comply with evacuation orders. The percentage of the population willing to evacuate will generally increase as a threat becomes more obvious or seems more serious to the population.
- Many residents who are not at risk and who are not in designated evacuation zones will also evacuate; this variable is difficult to quantify and accurately estimate, but has been observed in many past emergencies that required evacuation. This unknown number

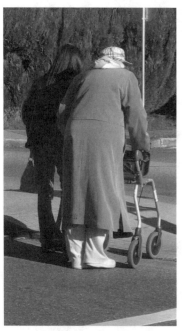

**Figure 7-1** EMS agencies must accommodate patients requiring assistance when preplanning for evacuation.

of residents complicates traffic planners' efforts to accurately estimate the saturation point of evacuation routes.

- Some residents will refuse to evacuate, no matter the risk of staying.
- Some owners of companion animals will refuse to evacuate unless they are allowed to take their animals with them. Service animals should be taken by their users during an evacuation.
- In most emergencies, the majority of evacuees will seek shelter with family, friends, or commercial accommodations rather than public shelters.
- Most evacuees will use their personal vehicles to evacuate. Some residents do not have their own vehicles. Nonambulatory residents may require lifting and moving assistance or transportation via stretcher in order to evacuate.

**Table 7-1** Local Government Responsibilities During Evacuation

**Chief Elected Official**

| | |
|---|---|
| • Make the recommendation that citizens evacuate when appropriate | • Approve release of evacuation-related warnings, instructions, and other emergency information |
| • Coordinate efforts with other local governments that may be affected | |

**Emergency Manager**

| | |
|---|---|
| • Direct the opening of emergency shelters and mass-care facilities | • Direct relocation of essential resources that are at risk to safer areas |
| • Identify risk areas in proximity to the incident site and determine protective actions for residents in those areas | • Develop/maintain evacuation planning information for known risk areas including population and evacuation routes |
| • Review evacuation plans of special facilities and determine possible needs for evacuation support | • Select suitable evacuation routes based on conditions |
| • Obtain and assign transportation resources | • Control movement of evacuees |

**Law Enforcement**

| | |
|---|---|
| • Make recommendations on evacuation route(s) to the emergency operations center (EOC) | • Protect property in evacuated areas and limit access to those areas |
| • Provide traffic control | • Protect, secure, and/or relocate prisoners |
| • Coordinate law enforcement activities with other emergency and law enforcement (LE) agencies | • Provide information on traffic and status of evacuation routes to public information officer (PIO) |
| • Assist in warning the public | |

**Emergency Medical Services**

| | |
|---|---|
| • Maintain transportation resource staging and accountability area; track and dispatch resources | • Monitor evacuation of hospitals and skilled-care facilities; coordinate evacuation assistance if needed |
| • Assist in evacuating the aged, handicapped, or other special needs groups | • Maintain communications with facilities to determine best destination for patients |
| • Assist in warning the public | • Request/recommend transportation resources from EOC |

*continues*

**Table 7-1** (Continued)

**Special Facility Operators**

| | |
|---|---|
| • Close and supervise evacuation of their facilities | • Coordinate transportation for evacuees and en route medical/security support |
| • Disseminate public information to advise relatives and the public on facility and patient status | • Request emergency assistance from local government if other assistance cannot be obtained |
| • Ensure facility personnel are trained and aware of evacuation procedures | • Arrange for use of suitable host facilities |

*Source:* Data from Kanawha Putnam Emergency Planning Committee, *Kanawha Putnam Emergency Management Plan* (Annex A04, "Evacuation"), Charlestown, WV, 2006.

## Hazard-Specific Evacuation Planning

It is imperative for EMS and emergency management staff to collaborate on advance planning for certain hazard-specific evacuation scenarios such as:

- Hazardous materials risk areas and major highways, railroads, ports, transfer facilities, and other transportation infrastructure where a hazardous materials incident is likely
- Hazardous manufacturing facilities
- Flooding and hurricane evacuation areas (predicted by flood zone maps and storm surge prediction maps)
- Areas where previous evacuations have occurred due to severe weather or other natural events

Hazard-specific annexes should be developed for each situation for inclusion in the local emergency management plan. Each possible situation should be evaluated and analyzed for:

- Impact areas for known hazards
- Population within impact area
- Homes or facilities with nonambulatory persons (eg, bariatric, technology-dependent, and mentally or physically challenged populations) who will require assistance
- Potential evacuation routes

## Planning for Special Facilities

Hospitals, skilled care or nursing/rehabilitation facilities, and even correctional centers will have some residents who require assistance during evacuation and should receive attention during the planning process. The vast majority of these facilities either through regulation or accreditation standards are required to have their own emergency plans, including evacuation plans. The completeness and level of detail in these plans may vary widely, as well as the frequency with which they are exercised.

The best-case scenario for special facilities is to evacuate all residents to like facilities outside of the emergency area. Planning for evacuation and coordinating with like facilities is the responsibility of the facility operator. A key component of EMS preplanning is interacting with these special facilities on a regular basis. EMS can assist the facility operators in maintaining and updating their emergency plans and can provide specific recommendations that will make the plans more effective. EMS planners can assist facility managers with planning for contracts with private ambulance services that can be executed during an emergency and provide guidance on the number of staff members and supplies that should be evacuated with each patient. This interaction will also help EMS and emergency management keep emergency plans current with an accurate number of patients in each facility that may require assistance. Emergency planning interaction can occur on an annual or semi-annual basis when EMS and/or fire officials visit special facilities for their normal preplanning reviews and fire inspections.

The challenge for EMS and local government will come in short-notice or no-notice evacuation situations when the facility operator may not be able to quickly execute emergency transportation contracts or when an emergency affects a large geographic area that includes like facilities in the evacuation plan.

# Preplanned Transportation Resources

It is helpful to have a preplanned list of potential transportation resources prior to an emergency evacuation. EMS agencies or the municipal government should contact government and nonprofit organizations about potential resources during the planning process and create mutual aid agreements (MAAs). Private, for-profit organizations that will require reimbursement should be engaged based on their willingness to enter into short-term, emergency contracts. The municipal government's finance or contracting department can create generic contracts that can be executed quickly in an emergency. Municipal emergency planners or the EMS agency should maintain periodic contact with transportation resources, and update the MAAs and renew contracts on at least an annual basis.

## Resources Subject to Local Planning and Preparation

Resources such as municipal EMS agencies, private and hospital-based ambulance services, para-transit vehicles, buses, aircraft, and military aircraft located outside the predicted disaster area should be included in local planning and preparation.

### Municipal EMS Agencies

Other EMS agencies can be expected to provide assistance, but the presence and status of MAAs must be verified. EMS agencies that the locality does not normally work with because of distance and geography may be a valuable resource in an emergency precisely because of distance and geography since they are outside of the disaster area. Interagency support may be covered by a statewide mutual aid agreement or multi-state compact. If not, formal MAAs should be negotiated and implemented.

### Private and Hospital-Based Ambulance Services

If several skilled care facilities in the area are evacuating at once, private ambulance services may be overwhelmed with the evacuation. Private and hospital-based services outside of the disaster area may provide assistance. The availability, willingness, and pricing of outside ambulance services should be investigated in advance, and appropriate emergency contracts and/or MAAs implemented in advance with the assistance of the municipal finance or purchasing department.

### Paratransit Vehicles

Paratransit (wheelchair) vehicles may be used for patients who have mobility constraints but do not necessarily need a medical attendant. Since paratransit vehicles come in multiple configurations from modified minivans up to full-size buses with wheelchair lifts, when asking for paratransit resources through the transportation unit or EOC, the requestor should specify the number of paratransit seats required versus the number of vehicles. Local and regional paratransit providers should be identified during the planning process, with contracts or MAA negotiated.

## Buses

Ambulatory patients may be moved via buses provided by a local school system, charter company, or transportation authority. Since bus drivers may not ordinarily be considered an emergency employee, identification and inclusion of these resources in the local emergency plan is essential; otherwise, bus drivers may evacuate with the rest of the community. Once identified, the following are planning considerations for utilizing bus resources for medical evacuation:

- *Agreements.* Negotiate and implement MAAs or contracts that address activation of the service, reimbursement, and workers' compensation for bus operators.
- *Communications.* Some mechanism of communications between the bus operator and the transportation unit is required in order to pass instructions to the operator on whether to return to a staging area, new pickup point, etc.
- *Medical staff.* The transportation unit supervisor may consider placing an EMT equipped with basic emergency supplies on the bus. For a bus convoy, consider adding an ambulance to accompany the convoy if one is available.

## Aircraft

Several considerations must be addressed in preplanning for aircraft utilization. EMS must determine whether a rotary wing or fixed wing aircraft will be needed. Rotary wing aircraft are more commonly known as helicopters; "fixed wing" refers to airplanes. Though this distinction seems simple, determining which type of aircraft is needed is important, as it allows EMS to incorporate the advantages of air transport into a preplan while minimizing its disadvantages.

Helicopters have the advantage of scene access, since they can enter vertically and drop down to a scene. There are several disadvantages, however, to helicopter use. Helicopters effectively accommodate a limited number of crew and patients. They also have weight limitations (patients, crew, and equipment) that ensure the aircraft can create lift to fly, range limitations, and altitude limitations during flight. The altitude limitation exists because helicopters are usually unpressurized, and in being unpressurized. As altitude increases, the partial pressure of oxygen falls, which can result in hypoxia of patients and staff.

Fixed-wing aircraft are usually able to carry more patients and crew, are usually pressurized (conditions on board will not effect the gases within the patient's body as much), and are able to operate at a significant range. The most significant disadvantage associated with airplane use is decreased access to a scene. As seen with the responses to Hurricanes Katrina and Rita, many patients were initially evacuated via helicopters and then transferred to airplanes for further evacuation.

Regardless of which aircraft is utilized, it is important to plan for equipment interoperability with EMS monitors and electrical systems, oxygen delivery, and stretcher/litter configuration when incorporating aircraft into an EMS preplan. The typical EMS stretcher will not fit into most aircraft; it may be necessary to transfer the patient before loading on the aircraft. This issue can be addressed at the time of initial transfer or evacuation, to minimize patient discomfort or injury.

## Military Aircraft

When planning for moving significant numbers of people, state or federal officials may coordinate for the use of military aircraft. Military aircraft have similar advantages and disadvantages as their civilian counterparts. Military aircraft are usually able to carry more patients and equipment due to their large size and payload.

## Resources That Require Coordination by the Emergency Operations Center

Resources requiring coordination by the EOC include the state ambulance task force, resources from the National Guard and Department of Defense (DoD), as well as Federal Emergency Management Agency (FEMA) ambulance contracts.

## State Ambulance Task Force

Many states organize ambulance task forces for mutual aid purposes. When local resources are overwhelmed, one or more task forces from outside the region can provide assistance. Task forces can also be mobilized and staged in advance for large-scale special events or evacuations. While organization varies from state to state, a task force normally includes four to five ambulances with crews and a supervisor. Agencies within the state that support ambulance task forces normally must provide task force members with training that includes incident command system (ICS) modules, national incident management system modules, and ambulance task force courses developed by the state. Depending on the state, an ambulance task force is requested from the state EOC by the local EOC. In some states, however, task forces are part of normal mutual aid cards or boxes and are requested in the same manner as other mutual aid.

## National Guard and DoD

Standard medical transportation vehicles with certified EMS providers are undoubtedly the best option for patient movement within a region, but severe catastrophes may warrant nonstandard vehicles to assist in patient movement due to an overwhelming number of patients, damage to regional EMS standard medical transport resources, or significant terrain challenges such as flooding. The National Guard and DoD may be requested to provide medical and nonmedical vehicles such as military ambulances, trucks, buses, and fixed-wing and rotary aircraft. A request for military assistance is processed through the state EOC to FEMA, which tasks the DoD with the request. Although there may be military resources local to the area, local military assets may not be free to be placed at the direct call of the local community because of the requirements of the base. It is not impossible to receive direct assistance, but prior coordination on what conditions would allow the local assets a quicker response may be negotiated with the local commander. Use of these resources will always be subject to higher military control.

The military is organized to support FEMA contingencies and can bring significant experience in logistics, transportation, medical care, and public-health capabilities. They can also provide specific assets to allow for continued response in an austere environment for extended time periods. Most of the time, military assets are self-contained and will not normally require assistance from other local agencies, except when requesting use of a space.

Since the mid-1990s, the military has gained significant experience in domestic and international disaster assistance. Although it may be somewhat intimidating to local agencies to work with military assets, it must be understood that the military's role is to support state or

---

### Massachusetts Ambulance Task Force System

The Commonwealth of Massachusetts in its mass-casualty preplanning uses the assumption that ambulance transportation may be required for 500 patients for every 1 million people. The Commonwealth has organized the state's EMS providers into 58 ambulance task forces, each of which contains five ambulances and a supervisor. Task forces may be advanced life support (ALS), basic life support (BLS), or a combination. Depending on local crew configuration, some task forces also deploy with ALS providers in separate vehicles. A total of about 290 ambulances are assigned to task forces.

When local and regional resources are exhausted, the incident commander requests a task force through the Mutual Aid District Control Center. The appropriate task force or forces are activated based on the running card via the National Warning System (NAWAS) phone system. Use of NAWAS also ensures that the Massachusetts Emergency Management Agency is aware of the task force activation and can effectively track resource availability statewide.

federal response activities. As a result, it is their duty to answer to whichever level ultimately requested their assistance.

### FEMA Ambulance Contract

In 2007, FEMA awarded the American Medical Response (AMR) a contract to provide supplemental ambulance service to communities experiencing disaster conditions. The primary contract covers the Gulf coast area (zone 1) and Atlantic coast area (zone 2). Contract options may be exercised to provide support to the rest of the continental United States. Utilizing AMR resources and a network of subcontractors, the contract allows a maximum deployment in each zone of 300 ground ambulances, 25 air ambulances, and paratransit vehicles capable of transporting 3,500 people. The contract has been activated a number of times since it was awarded for hurricane evacuation and in support of the January 2009 inauguration of President Barack Obama. The ambulance contract is a Federal resource and must be requested via the State EOC.

## National Disaster Medical System

According to FEMA, the *National Response Framework* (*NRF*) presents the guiding principles that enable all response partners to prepare for and provide a unified national response to disasters and emergencies. It establishes a comprehensive, national, all-hazards approach to domestic incident response. The NRF's Emergency Support Function 8 (ESF-8) is led by the Department of Health and Human Services (DHHS) with the assistance of 13 other agencies. ESF-8 provides four principle types of services: medical services, mental health services, environmental health services, and preventative health services. The NDMS provides the federal response in support of medical and mental health services.

The DoD and Department of Veterans Affairs (VA) manage a system of 70 NDMS Federal Coordinating Centers (FCCs) around the country. Each of these centers is in close proximity to a large airport for air transportation access; is in or near a major metropolitan area with a number of hospitals in close proximity; and has the staff and other resources to manage a patient reception area (PRA)/patient distribution area (PDA). Approximately 2,000 federal and nonfederal hospitals voluntarily maintain affiliation with the NDMS, offering about 100,000 patient beds.

Under the NDMS patient movement concept, the system is activated when a community's health care resources are overwhelmed. The local community requests NDMS support via the local EOC through the state EOC to the global patient movement requirement center (GPMRC) at Scott Air Force Base, IL. The appropriate military transportation resources are matched to the need and dispatched to the requesting community's local airport. The closest FCC assists the overwhelmed community's hospital(s) by coordinating transportation from the affected hospital(s) to the airport and by establishing a mobile aeromedical staging facility (MASF) at the airport. MASF staff prepare the patients for transport by exchanging hospital equipment for air-worthy substitutes, verifying patient data and medical records with the manifest, and monitoring and treating patients until loaded on the aircraft.

Meanwhile, an FCC is chosen to receive the evacuated patients and is activated and ordered to establish a PRA/PDA. The receiving PRA will have activated the necessary staff to receive patients. Once the aircraft arrives at the PRA/PDA, patients are unloaded, assessed, and retriaged.

### National Disaster Medical System

The NDMS is a public–private partnership created to address two main medical contingencies in the US: A large natural or manmade disaster that results in overwhelming casualties, and the treatment and movement of large numbers of military casualties that overwhelm the DoD and the VA. The DHHS provides the on-scene medical care component of the NDMS through multiple disaster medical assistance teams. The DoD provides patient movement capabilities using military transportation assets and a network of federal coordinating hospitals. The DoD and the VA coordinate definitive care through a network of military, veterans affairs, and civilian hospitals.

Local transportation resources distribute the patients to participating NDMS hospitals that have been prenotified by the receiving FCC.

The mass movement of hospital and other patients in the aftermath of Hurricane Katrina was the first full-scale activation and use of the NDMS system. A C-130 Hercules military transport aircraft is capable of carrying up to 74 litter patients at its maximum configuration; typically no more than 50 are carried due to difficult litter access and height issues on the aircraft. Additionally, usually no more than six critical patients can be carried per flight due to limitations on available, trained military aeronautical medical staff. The challenge and likely role for EMS in NDMS patient movement scenarios is an FCC receiving 50 litter patients at one time. Planning the transportation function for an NDMS PRA is much like running transportation at a mass-casualty incident (MCI), with the bonus of having some length of time to alert and prepare resources.

The receiving FCC coordinates staff for patient care and assessment, litter bearers, and patient administration and tracking. Ambulance transportation is the most likely role for the local EMS system, including coordinating mutual aid and private transport resources to assist, if needed. Planning considerations for managing transportation for an NDMS PRA/PDA include:

- *Awareness of agency management and providers.* Management and EMS planners should participate in NDMS FCC meetings and exercises.
- *Standard operating procedures (SOPs) and protocols.* The EMS agency should create and implement an SOP or protocol that addresses the agency's responsibilities at the PRA/PDA. Like an MCI, certain equipment and supplies will be necessary to provide a smooth transportation unit:
  - Base station medical radios and antenna
  - Patient tracking forms
  - Triage tags agreed on by the EMS agency and FCC
  - Preprinted maps, directions, and phone numbers for NDMS receiving hospitals
  - ICS 211 forms for tracking transportation staff and resources
  - Mechanism for fueling and replacing onboard oxygen on ambulances
- *MAAs and/or MOUs.* These should be updated and edited to reflect participation by mutual aid partners in the NDMS PDA transportation function. An FCC's regional NDMS hospital network may take mutual aid providers out of their normal service areas, and this should be addressed. The NDMS covers routine ambulance transportation costs, so billing and reimbursement information should be addressed with mutual aid providers in advance.
- *Communications and status.* Since the regional NDMS hospital network may take transport resources outside normal radio range and multiple mutual aid partners may be involved in the patient movement, communications issues should be addressed in advance. In any case after delivering a patient, transporting ambulances must contact the PDA to advise of their status and receive instructions regarding returning to their home base or returning to the PDA for another patient.
- *Reimbursement of mutual aid transportation providers.* NDMS reimburses ambulance services for patient transportation, generally at or above normal Medicaid billing levels. Invoices for transportation services provided for each patient are submitted to the Department of Homeland Security using guidance and specific mission-tasking information provided by the FCC.

## Incident Management

The incident command organization managing large-scale patient movement should include a transportation unit. Since the ICS is scalable and flexible, both the overall command organization as well as the transportation unit can be built to accommodate the event, from the evacuation of a single hospital that experiences a fire, to an entire geographic region being evacuated due to an approaching hurricane. All transportation resource requests should be funneled through the transportation unit to ensure the most appropriate resource is dispatched and utilized. Transportation units serving large geographic areas may further organize resources into strike teams or divisions based on geography and workload (see **Figure 7-2**). Deployments, mileage, and expenses must be documented and forwarded to the finance branch.

Planning considerations for the transportation unit supervisor include traffic routes, ambulance exchange points, logistic support along evacuation routes, communications with the transport unit, and support for out-of-area units.

### Traffic Routes

For an isolated incident, the best travel routes may be dictated by the incident commander, emergency management officials, or a hazard-specific preplan or emergency plan annex. For large-scale evacuations due to weather events and other natural disasters, travel routes will likely be dictated by state emergency management or highway officials. Some traffic management plans involve reversing traffic direction in order to accommodate more traffic; in other words, the interstate highway that normally carries inbound traffic to a community may have some or all lanes reversed in order to double the capacity of outbound traffic. EMS planners must collaborate with traffic and emergency management officials on an effective route to allow ambulances and other resources to return for subsequent trips.

### Ambulance Exchange Points

Ambulance exchange points are locations where patients can be transferred from one mode of transportation to another. During a long-distance evacuation or patient movement it might be more feasible to "hand off" a patient to another EMS agency to continue the transport after 150 to 200 miles or so. An NDMS patient debarkation airport or other location where an ambulance patient is moved to or from an aircraft (or any other mode of transportation) is another example of an ambulance exchange point. If ambulance exchange points are established, there should be medical support and patient movement staff available, as well as some method of crew and patient accountability as patient transfers take place and ambulance crews depart to return to the scene for further assignments.

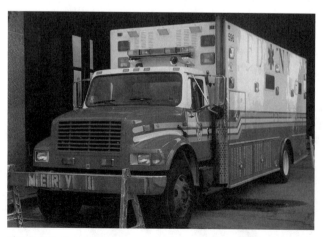

**Figure 7-2** Many large EMS systems deploy specialized MCI units or mobile emergency room vehicles (as shown here) that are able to treat dozens of patients on the scene.

### Logistics Along Evacuation Routes

Access control points along planned evacuation routes may prevent traffic from exiting a highway. EMS system planners must work with traffic officials so that ambulance operators have knowledge of where they can exit and return to the highway if needed. Vehicles break down; the EMS system that normally utilizes a municipal wrecker and fuel farm must plan for the eventuality of a breakdown or the need to purchase fuel when the ambulance is operating well outside of the normal municipal boundaries during an evacuation. Emergency credit cards and written agreements with other municipalities along the evacuation route are two methods that can be used for vehicle-related needs.

Oxygen is a finite resource; the transportation unit dispatcher and ambulance crews must collaborate on matching the best transport resource for each patient.

Extra portable tanks should be considered for long-distance trips. Weather event planning should emphasize careful attention to onboard oxygen tank levels in the days and hours leading up to a planned weather-related evacuation.

## Communications With the Transport Unit

During evacuation operations outside of the normal response area, radio communications may be impossible due to distance. Any statewide radio networks including med-radio networks should be considered for communications with the transporting unit. Preplanning for this eventuality includes knowledge of the available communications infrastructure and state communications plans, proper programming of mobile radios, and employee awareness and training. Cell phones or landline telephones may be considered as a backup communications method with the under-standing that the event that caused the evacuation in the first place may also affect the cell and landline phone systems. Ambulance operators must have some method of reporting in to the transportation unit once their transport is complete in order to receive instructions to return for another transport or to shelter where they are.

## Support for Out-of-Area Mutual Aid

Communications capabilities of agencies with which MAAs exist should be identified in advance. If mutual aid responders are to report directly to a specific location to receive patients, it is helpful to specify what radio channel will be used when requesting their response. If mutual aid units are to report to a staging area, the staging manager should provide arriving units with communications information.

Areas prone to natural or weather events such as earthquakes or hurricanes should consider building and maintaining a cache of portable radios to be available for mutual aid resources. Agencies should also be prepared to offer normal EMS logistics support including fuel and vehicle maintenance, oxygen refills, and supply replenishment.

Local maps and maps of the evacuation routes should also be available for out-of-area mutual aid resources. Another consideration is exchanging a local EMT with an EMT from an out-of-area resource.

# Standard of Care and EMS System Saturation

While unpleasant to consider, it is important to recognize during the planning process that there may come a point when the EMS system is saturated to the point that it can no longer maintain the standard of care it normally delivers. Increased reliance on mutual aid and private ambulance services for disaster transportation waters down the system's oversight of quality and standards. A normally all-ALS system may have no choice but to utilize BLS crews. Mutual aid services may not offer the interventions and treatment modalities normally provided by the community's EMS system. For planning purposes, it may be helpful to review the following progressive saturation scenarios, overlay the specifics of the EMS system, and consider specific actions that should be implemented to compensate for fewer available transport and treatment resources.

### Moderate Saturation Level

- Local units are capable of responding to all requests for service without change to the normal level of patient care provided.
  - Hospital emergency departments are extremely busy with long patient wait times.
  - Patient turnover to hospital staff is delayed.
  - Full emergency departments result in increased diversion to hospitals that are farther away.

- Transport, turnover, and out-of-service times per unit are increased.
- Call volume is abnormally high.
  - Response times are increased, and low-priority calls are stacked pending an available unit.

### Substantial Saturation Level

- System is substantially impacted; standard of care starts to be impacted by nontraditional patient destination, increased response times, and mixture of outside mutual aid resources.
  - Hospital emergency departments cannot absorb all seriously ill/injured patients. Some seriously ill/injured patients must be transported outside the normal cachement area.
  - Minor injuries and illnesses are diverted to clinics, urgent care centers, physician offices, or held on scene at MCIs.
  - Local, regional, or state disaster declaration or state-of-emergency declaration is made or anticipated.
  - EMS transport resources are consistently delayed, even for high priority calls.

### Critical Saturation Level or Locally Declared Disaster

- System is seriously impacted and unable to respond to all calls for service. Austere treatment at auxiliary sites such as temporary disaster medical centers, shelters, and on scene at MCIs must be implemented.
  - Emergency departments, physician offices, clinics, urgent care centers, and other facilities cannot meet demand and see all patients; supplies and medications may run low.
  - Large numbers of patients converge on medical facilities.
    - All local and mutual aid transport resources are exhausted pending state or out-of-state assistance.
    - EMS transport resources are significantly delayed. Some low-priority calls for service do not receive an EMS response.

It is important that EMS agency heads and planners recognize and understand limitations on normal standard of care during disaster operations and address in advance what mitigations the system will allow in order to operate at maximum efficiency. Some questions that should be considered by the EMS system are:

- Will reserve ambulances that are not fully equipped be placed into service as transport units?
- Does the agency have a policy or protocol that allows suspension of normal destination plans?
- If the agency operates an all-electronic patient care report system, is there a paper-based backup plan that can be utilized by mutual aid resources and agency resources that do not have access to mobile data terminals or other computer systems during disaster operations?
- How will the agency staff alternative transport resources such as buses?
- What is the minimum provider level and staffing mix that the agency will utilize to staff licensed EMS transport vehicles?
- If the EMS system performs interfacility and other routine transports, is there a policy or protocol in place to prioritize transports that are absolutely necessary and cancel or reschedule the rest?
- Is there a medical dispatch system in place that effectively triages and prioritizes 9-1-1 calls (see **Figure 7-3**)?

- Is there a dispatch protocol in place that allows dispatchers to deny service to low-priority callers, instead advising the caller of resource status and offering preapproved medical instructions?
- Is there a policy or protocol to dispatch first responders only, to confirm the need for transport resources or ALS care, prior to sending an ambulance or ALS resources during periods of critical saturation? Are responders prepared to deny service to low-acuity patients?
- Is there a plan for public service announcements that offer instructions on proper use of 9-1-1 and available medical facilities?
- Is there a plan for public service announcements that include reminders for residents to try to assist their neighbors who need help or who do not have their own means of evacuation?
- Is the EMS system medical director involved in the development and approval of all policies and protocols that impact standard of care?

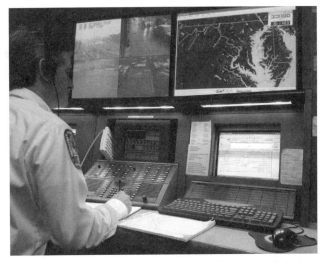

**Figure 7-3** The dispatcher will coordinate the entire rescue effort, while ensuring effective prioritization of 9-1-1 calls.

While it is generally accepted that the normal standard of care may not be available for all patients during disaster operations, there should be logical and medically necessary rationale for how care is rationed during an emergency. For risk management and liability purposes, it is essential that the EMS system utilizes some standard [emergency medical dispatching (EMD) priority dispatch cards, protocols, regional mass-casualty plan, etc] method of triage and prioritization and that the method chosen is clinically prudent and acceptable, as evidenced by the involvement and approval of the system medical director.

## Preplanning to Facilitate Effective Evacuation

When planning for large-scale medical transportation needs, planners must consider both scenarios that provide some warning to emergency officials and sudden events with little or no advance notice. Whether it is a single hospital that experiences a fire or an entire community including hospitals and other licensed care facilities affected by a natural disaster, the primary role of EMS will likely be facilitating and coordinating the mass patient movement effort. Preplanning is essential both at the facility level with its particular patient population and on the community and regional levels with analysis in advance of available resources, logistics needs, evacuation routes, and other characteristics. The transportation component of an incident management system must be adequately staffed with competent leaders who are aware of the available local, state, and federal resources and know how to access them.

EMS systems that serve highly populated areas should be prepared to support the National Disaster Medical System's patient movement function in order to evacuate patients out of the area or to receive and distribute patients from other parts of the country.

Inundation of EMS resources may result in a degradation of the community's normal standard of care; mechanisms to prioritize calls

### Preplanning Practices

Evacuation has some significant risks involved, even when the operation is properly planned. At the scene of an incident, EMS personnel should think carefully and consider all options before proceeding with a full-scale evacuation.

for service and conserve resources for true needs must be prepared. Effective planning for large-scale transportation needs requires an organized approach to incident management and attention to and familiarity with a range of written plans and procedures from local protocols, preplanning documents, and emergency plans to state-level plans and the NRF.

## Selected References

American Medical Response: *Overview of FEMA/AMR National Disaster Emergency Medical Services*; March 9, 2009 revision. http://www.amr.net/Disaster-Response/AMR-Disaster-Response-Team-References-and-Resource.aspx. Accessed December 1, 2009

Centers for Disease Control and Prevention: *Chemical Agents: Facts About Sheltering in Place*. US Department of Health and Human Services; August, 16, 2006.

Emergency Medical Services Administrators Association of California: *Coordination of Prehospital Emergency Services*; draft paper, undated.

Franco, C, Toner, E, et al.: The national disaster medical system: Past, present, and suggestions for the future. *Biosecurity and Bioterrorism* 2007;5:4, 319–325.

Kanawha Putnam Emergency Planning Committee: *Kanawha Putnam Emergency Management Plan* (Annex A04, "Evacuation"). Charlestown, WV; 2006.

Knouss, RF: National disaster medical system. *Public Health Reports*, supplement 2, volume 116. Rockville, MD: US Department of Heath and Human Services, Office of Emergency Preparedness/Federal Emergency Management Agency; 2001.

McGovern, JE: Casualty evacuation and patient movement. *Special Operations Medical Support*. Lenexa, KS: National Association of Emergency Physicians; 2009.

National Disaster Medical System (NDMS): *Federal Coordinating Center Guide*. Washington, D.C.: Department of Health and Human Services; 2006.

State of Texas Emergency Management, Governor's Division of Emergency Management: *2007 Hurricane Dean After Action Report*; November 26, 2007.

United States Department of Homeland Security: Mass evacuation: Developing a contraflow plan. *Lessons Learned Information Sharing*. https://www.llis.dhs.gov/index.do.

United States Department of Homeland Security: Mass evacuation: Triage units at embarkation points. *Lessons Learned Information Sharing*. https://www.llis.dhs.gov/index.do.

United States Department of Homeland Security: *National Response Framework*; January, 2008. http://www.dhs.gov/files/programs/editorial_0566.shtm. Accessed December 1, 2009.

# Chapter 8

# Shelters and Mass Care

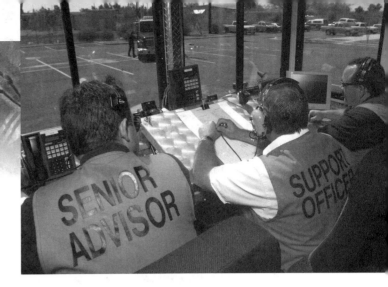

## Introduction to Shelters and Mass Care

Natural and manmade emergencies may result in communities opening one or more temporary shelters to provide protection and lodging for displaced members of the community. Responsibility for the planning and operation of shelters varies widely based on the size of the community, organization of local government, and availability of government and private sector resources and agencies equipped to operate shelters. In some communities emergency medical services (EMS) may have no responsibility at all for assisting with shelter operations, while in others, EMS has a much larger role. From a planning perspective, it is important to be aware of the EMS agency's responsibilities as set forth in the local emergency plan, and to have an agency plan or procedure that addresses those responsibilities and effectively considers exactly how the EMS agency will conduct operations once shelters are opened.

The opening of emergency shelters and other mass-care operations indicates a significant local emergency. The relocation and sheltering of large numbers of citizens is a tremendous undertaking that a single local agency is unlikely to be able to perform by itself. The opening, staffing, and operation of shelters normally involves multiple agencies of local government including emergency management, public health, public safety, and social services, as well as nonprofit entities such as the American Red Cross, amateur radio clubs, and the faith community. Because of the varying capabilities and resources each entity brings to the table, the complexities of interagency communications, record keeping, and finance procedures, it is essential to thoroughly preplan these operations, test the plans with exercises, and carefully evaluate exercise and real event results to modify and improve the plans accordingly.

## Legal Authority

Because of the large-scale nature of events that result in shelter operations, communities often receive reimbursement for emergency operations from the state, which may receive reimbursement from the federal government. The frequently used term disaster actually has legal meaning in the

---

### Preplanning Practices

**EMS in the Local Plan**

*Determine* where your EMS agency fits into existing community emergency plans: Is the agency tasked with specific responsibilities when shelters are opened?

*Determine* whether your agency can actually fulfill its requirements under the plan with existing resources.

*Develop* an internal procedure guiding the agency through the specific steps required to fulfill its responsibilities under the local emergency plan.

*Implement* mutual aid agreements (MAAs) and interservice support agreements (ISSAs) necessary to ensure that the EMS agency can meet its obligations under the plan while maintaining normal response capability.

emergency management community. A fire that destroys a long-time, locally owned business on Main Street may indeed be a disaster for the business owners, but the community at large is not significantly impacted and large-scale local government resources are not expended to compensate the owners. If a fire originates in a local business and burns an entire city block, destroying several other businesses and forcing the relocation of dozens of tenants of a ruined apartment building, chances are the community will bring to bear many more resources to support the affected citizens. In this instance, the town's mayor may declare a state of emergency and ask the governor for a local disaster declaration.

---

### Legal Authority Definitions

*Disaster* (federal definition): Any hurricane, tornado, storm, flood, high-water, wind-driven water, tidal wave, tsunami, earthquake, volcanic eruption, landslide, mudslide, snowstorm, drought, fire, explosion, or other catastrophe in any part of the United States that requires federal emergency assistance to supplement state and local efforts to save lives and protect public health and safety or to avert or lessen the threat of a major disaster.

*Disaster declaration*: Formal declaration of disaster conditions performed by the governor or president. Enables state and federal disaster funds and resources to flow to the disaster area.

*Local emergency*: The duly proclaimed existence of conditions of disaster or of extreme peril to the safety of persons and property within the territorial limits of a county, city and county, or city, caused by such conditions as air pollution, fire, flood, storm, epidemic, riot, earthquake, or other conditions that are, or are likely to be, beyond the control of the services, personnel, equipment, and facilities of a political subdivision and require the combined forces of other political subdivisions to combat.

*State of emergency*: The duly proclaimed existence of conditions of disaster or of extreme peril for the safety of persons and property within the state caused by such conditions as air pollution, fire, flood, storm, epidemic, riot, drought, sudden and severe energy shortage, plant or animal infection or disease, the governor's warning of an earthquake or volcanic prediction, or an earthquake, or other conditions, which conditions, by reason of their magnitude, are or are likely to be beyond the control of the services, personnel, equipment, and facilities of any single county, city and county, or city, and require the combined forces of a mutual aid region or regions to combat.

*Major disaster*: Any natural catastrophe (including any hurricane, tornado, storm, high water, wind-driven water, tidal wave, tsunami, earthquake, volcanic eruption, landslide, mudslide, snowstorm, or drought) or, regardless of cause, any fire, flood, or explosion, in any part of the United States, which in the determination of the president causes damage of sufficient severity and magnitude to warrant major disaster assistance to supplement the efforts and available resources of states, local governments, and disaster relief organizations in alleviating the damage, loss, hardship, or suffering.

---

The declaration of a state of emergency allows the municipal government to temporarily suspend certain procedures and implement rules and policies necessary to protect the public safety and preserve property and infrastructure. For instance, in order for local government to tear down a derelict building, it normally must first go through the legal process of condemnation, have funds appropriated by the city council to pay for the demolition, then advertise and solicit competitive bids for the project. By declaring a state of emergency for the example above where a city block was destroyed by fire, the normal financial appropriations rules and legal advertising, public notice, and competitive bid process are suspended, and the government may quickly contract with a demolition or construction company to raze damaged structures to prevent their collapse and rid the community of the hazard of structurally unsound buildings.

Likewise, a disaster declaration by the governor allows state agencies to temporarily suspend certain rules and procedures in order to quickly allow aid to flow into a damaged community. In the example above, the governor's disaster declaration may allow affected residents to receive unemployment benefits without the typical application process and waiting period, and reimbursement to the local government for the costs of providing shelter to affected residents or the replacement of firefighting equipment damaged during the incident.

Funding and reimbursement for emergency operations during declared emergencies and disasters may be critical in assisting recovery efforts in a community; the planning process for these emergencies must address documentation and record keeping in order for agencies to be properly reimbursed. The mechanism for reimbursement is usually announced by the lead agency after the disaster or incident is well-established or, in many instances, either immediately after the incident or as units or agencies are released from assignment.

The Robert T. Stafford Disaster Relief and Emergency Assistance Act directs the provision of technical assistance to the states for the development of comprehensive emergency plans, provides grants for plan development and maintenance, and allows federal loans and grants to states, businesses, and individuals. This federal statute allows federal agencies to provide resources and assistance including medicine, food, and other consumables in support of state or local disaster relief efforts. The act also allows the direct reimbursement of state and local government and nonprofit agencies. The federal share of disaster relief costs is generally 75% or more of the total, with state government responsible for the remainder. The Stafford Act also provides for the reimbursement of states for costs incurred by activating and utilizing the National Guard and overtime costs for local and state employees during disasters.

State laws and regulations detail state-level authority and responsibility during emergencies. State laws dictate the responsibilities and authority of the governor, state agencies, and local government, and they detail the specific processes for state-level disaster declarations and states of emergency.

Local ordinances designate the government officials that are responsible for emergency management in communities. Ordinances enacted by the city or town council or county board of supervisors or commissioners may authorize the city or county manager to enter into MAAs, designate the local emergency manager, and grant authority to issue local emergency declarations and activate the emergency operations center, among other things. When a nongovernment organization (NGO; such as the local American Red Cross chapter) has significant responsibility within the local emergency plan, the organization's role may be codified by an ordinance that specifies who has the authority to request assistance from the organization and the process for financial reimbursement.

---

### Nongovernment Organization

An NGO is an agency or association that serves a public purpose that is not related to or created by government. NGOs frequently cooperate with and assist government, particularly in areas of social services and disaster relief. Examples include faith-based organizations such as churches, fraternal and service organizations such as Boy Scouts, Jaycees, and the American Legion, and humanitarian organizations like the American Red Cross and Salvation Army.

## Legal Agreements

By definition, a disaster is an event that overwhelms the local ability to mitigate its associated hazards. In dealing with managing a large event, it may be necessary for an EMS agency or municipality to request additional assistance from neighboring jurisdictions, including regional and state agencies. Usually, local assistance comes in the form of MAAs with neighboring jurisdictions such as neighboring EMS agencies, fire departments, or law enforcement agencies.

When requesting assistance within the jurisdiction from nontraditional responders (eg, transportation, public health, parks, water, and sanitation), ISSAs are utilized for requesting, managing, and defining assistance.

### Mutual Aid Agreements

MAAs formally define the relationships between two or more agencies or municipalities and the support those organizations will provide to each other when requested. EMS is normally accustomed to MAAs that allow EMS services and fire departments in neighboring jurisdictions to cover emergency calls, but many local governments and government agencies utilize MAAs for other services. Neighboring county social services agencies may enter into an MOU to allow case management, counseling, and other services across jurisdictional boundaries. Local health departments may enter into such agreements to allow the sharing of vaccine or laboratory services. Well-written MAAs normally specify that aid provided under the agreement is "cost neutral," or specifies a reimbursement method. MAAs should also cover liability issues such as the responsibility for reimbursement for equipment damaged or lost during a mutual aid response, and responsibility of worker's compensation payments and death benefits for employees of one local government who are injured while performing work for another local government under an MAA.

### Interservice Support Agreements

ISSAs are a type of MAA used by sister agencies within the same local government structure. Most department and agency heads within local government report directly to the city or county manager or head elected official (depending on local government organization). ISSAs become important when one agency needs the services of another in the absence of a declared emergency or when a local government service does not answer directly to the city manager. For example, a locality that includes the county and several incorporated towns and cities may create an authority to run its sanitation, public works, or utility services. An authority is typically managed by an executive board made up of local government managers or elected officials from each of the jurisdictions it serves. The head of the public works authority likely does not answer directly to any of the local governments. If a fire or EMS agency needed the services of the public works authority on a weekend or after hours to provide a portable generator or to execute a contract for portable toilets at a scene where fire and EMS will be working for an extended period, the authority may insist that the fire or EMS agency reimburse it for overtime and fuel for the generator or contract costs for the toilets before it responds. The public works authority may further have to receive authorization to expend overtime from its head official, delaying the response. An ISSA, like other MAAs, lays out specific authority and procedures in advance, so that local government agencies can support each other with a minimum of delay.

### Statewide MAAs

The process of negotiating, maintaining, and updating MAAs can be cumbersome and time-consuming. Most localities maintain detailed MAAs with neighboring communities with whom they routinely share response resources, but not with communities located some distance away with whom they seldom interact. Many states facilitate a statewide MAA. By becoming a signatory to the statewide agreement, local governments gain the benefit of a basic, legal framework with other localities within the state that are party to the agreement. In the instance of a large-scale emergency, the localities have a much larger pool of intrastate resources available to them, even without the formal declaration of a disaster or state of emergency.

### Emergency Management Assistance Compacts

EMACs are nationwide, interstate MAAs administered by the National Association of Emergency Managers and chartered by Congress. While states often have existing agreements governing everything from emergency response to professional licensing with other contiguous states with whom they routinely share services, law enforcement operations, and trade, the EMAC provides a "master" MAA with other states and territories within the United States. EMACs may be used with or without a concurrent federal response or disaster declaration. The compact addresses issues of legal liability, workers' compensation, and reimbursement, as well as other administrative and legal issues.

> **Emergency Management Assistance Compact**
>
> A congressionally ratified organization that provides form and structure to interstate mutual aid. Through EMACs, a disaster-affected state can request and receive assistance from other member states quickly and efficiently, resolving two key issues up front: liability and reimbursement.

## Shelter Operations

An EMS agency's responsibility to shelter operations may be as simple as responding to 9-1-1 calls while the shelter is open, to providing 24-hour primary care services for shelter residents. In order to effectively plan for EMS integration into shelter operations, EMS leaders must understand the basics of shelter operations.

The local emergency manager typically determines when shelters must be opened. In rural or small communities, the emergency manager may not be a full-time government employee, but a collateral duty assigned to the fire chief, sheriff, or other local official. Once the determination has been made that emergency shelter is needed, the emergency manager and local agencies responsible for shelter operation determine how many shelters will be required and which shelter locations are most appropriate for the need.

Many communities rely on the American Red Cross as the primary resource in shelter operations. The American Red Cross is an NGO, but is chartered by Congress to: "Carry out a system of national and international relief in time of peace, and apply that system in mitigating the suffering caused by pestilence, famine, fire, floods, and other great national calamities, and to devise and carry out measures for preventing those calamities…" The American Red Cross is uniquely qualified to organize and operate emergency shelters because of its experience and history in disaster relief operations, network of local, state, and international chapters and resources, and organized training modules in shelter operations. The American Red Cross maintains cadres of volunteers in various specialties who are available to carry out its disaster assistance mission. Other NGOs including the Salvation Army, Mennonite Disaster Services, and others may assist in operating local shelters. The American Red Cross is specifically tasked as a support agency with assigned functions listed in Emergency Support Function 6 (ESF 6), an annex of the National Response Framework (NRF). The functions are mass care, emergency assistance, housing, and human services.

Because of legal, political, or organizational issues and local availability of NGO disaster services in specific locations, some communities place a local government organization such as its health or human services department in charge of coordinating and operating emergency shelters. No matter which government agency or NGO is tasked with shelter operations, it must be legally designated as such by the local government.

> **Emergency Support Functions**
>
> Similar functions within the NRF are grouped into ESFs. There are 15 ESFs (see **Table 8-1**), each with an annex describing their roles, responsibilities, and responsible agencies in the NRF.

Likewise, states must designate the state-level organization for coordinating mass care within the state.

Once shelters to be opened are identified, the shelter team arrives and verifies that prestaged equipment caches are in place, or coordinates the movement of trailers containing needed commodities to the proper locations. Communications are established with the shelter branch coordinator or emergency operations center (EOC) by phone or radio. Amateur radio clubs often provide this service and may be integrated in the local emergency plan for this purpose. Once staff is in place and necessary supplies and equipment arrive, the shelter opens and begins receiving residents.

| Table 8-1 | Emergency Support Functions |
|---|---|
| ESF #1 | Transportation |
| ESF #2 | Communications |
| ESF #3 | Public works and engineering |
| ESF #4 | Firefighting |
| ESF #5 | Emergency management |
| ESF #6 | Mass care, emergency assistance, housing, and human services |
| ESF #7 | Logistics management and resource support |
| ESF #8 | Public health and medical services |
| ESF #9 | Search and rescue |
| ESF #10 | Oil and hazardous materials response |
| ESF #11 | Agriculture and natural awareness |
| ESF #12 | Energy |
| ESF #13 | Public safety and security |
| ESF #14 | Long-term community recovery |
| ESF #15 | External affairs |

Source: Data from the FEMA, *Emergency Support Function Annexes*, January 2008.

Upon arrival, residents are registered. The registration should include pre- and post-disaster addresses, names and ages of all family members, and any health concerns or special needs. The American Red Cross utilizes a standard shelter registration form. Communities may develop their own form, or even use 3- × 5-inch index cards. For safety and accountability purposes, most shelter managers implement a mandatory sign-in/sign-out process for all residents. Persons with suspected infectious diseases, persons who require advanced medical care or observation, and children with no parent or guardian present should be segregated away from the shelter's general population.

Depending on the length of time the shelter is anticipated to be in operation, status of local businesses, and safety and general condition of the surrounding area after a disaster, coordinated food services may be provided to shelter residents. Health care services may also be provided. Local EMS services, American Red Cross volunteer shelter nurses, local public health nurses, or other providers give basic primary care and referrals outside the shelter for more complicated needs. Generally, if a shelter is open for more than 48 to 72 hours, the local public health official may initiate assessment visits to assess current disease conditions, sanitation and cleanliness, and the need for mental and behavioral health counselors. Refrigeration may be needed for insulin and other medications.

Throughout shelter operations, reports are periodically provided to the shelter branch manager or EOC. Reports include shelter status, feeding operations status, medical incident, or health status. Upon conclusion of shelter activities, an after action report (AAR) is compiled and submitted.

## Mass-Care Shelter Staff

Whether operated by the American Red Cross, public health service, or other volunteer or government agency, the following are typical positions that are necessary at all mass-care shelters:

- *Shelter manager.* Overall manager at an individual shelter. Manages all operations and staff including volunteers. Keeps staff and evacuees updated on events. Reports to the shelter branch director.
- *Operations manager/assistant shelter manager.* (This position is sometimes staffed in large shelters.) The chief operating officer of the shelter, responsible for all aspects of shelter operations including registration of residents, traffic and security, resident assignment, segregation, and transfers.
- *Facilities.* The facilities technician may be part of the mobilized shelter team or an employee of the hosting facility (such as a school or other government building). Ensures that the facility and physical plant are capable of operating under emergency conditions. Keeps the shelter clean and functional. Coordinates with utilities, sanitation, and operates emergency power. Reports to shelter manager (or operations manager/assistant shelter manager at large shelters).
- *Medical technician.* Nurse, paramedic, or emergency medical technician that provides basic primary care services and first aid to residents. Assists residents with medication storage and administration. Determines when ill or injured residents must be transferred to a medical needs shelter or definitive care such as a hospital. May report to shelter manager or medical unit leader.
- *Case manager.* This position is normally a licensed social worker from the jurisdiction's social or community services department or a counselor or American Red Cross volunteer with special training. Evaluates residents to determine need for financial, mental health, or other support. Assists in coordinating care with primary care and specialty physicians, pharmacies, and other health services. Coordinates placement of evacuees in more suitable accommodations including family and health care facilities outside the disaster area. May report to shelter manager, medical unit, or community services/social work unit.
- *Communications.* Assists the team with maintaining contact with shelter branch director and the EOC. Operates telephones, radio, and computers as necessary to communicate and provide updates to incident command and request additional resources. This team member is often provided by a local amateur radio club or network. Reports to shelter manager (or operations manager/assistant shelter manager at large shelters).
- *Registration team.* Registers and logs all incoming and outgoing residents. The registration team may have health care providers that triage patients who are ill or injured, and make decisions on segregating residents into special areas for unaccompanied minors, patients with special medical needs, or infectious disease. The registration team leader reports to shelter manager (or operations manager/assistant shelter manager at large shelters).
- *General staff.* Shelter team staff members set up patient sleeping areas, issue comfort items, enforce shelter rules, and assist residents with any issues or problems that arise.
- *Logistics manager.* Ensures that the shelter has the resources that it needs to operate including equipment, supplies, and personnel. Accounts for equipment and supplies and orders needed resources. The logistics team may also coordinate food service. Reports to shelter manager (or operations manager/assistant shelter manager at large shelters).

# Plans

According to the NRF, the local senior elected or appointed official is responsible for ensuring the safety and welfare of community residents. State governments, specifically the governor, are responsible for public safety and welfare of residents within the state. It is the governor's responsibility to coordinate emergency actions among the many local governments and state agencies and to request outside assistance from other states or the federal government when needed.

When developing local emergency plans or agency standard operating procedures, a valuable concept to follow is that utilized by the NRF. The NRF has five key principles that together form the doctrine for an effective emergency plan:

- Engaged partnerships
- Tiered response
- Scalable, flexible, and adaptable response capabilities
- Unity of effort through unified command
- Readiness to act

Even the best planned, staffed, and equipped shelter is an austere environment when compared with most homes. The primary goal from the time the shelter doors open is to return occupants to their normal situations as soon as possible. Barring a return to normal, the goal is to relocate occupants into better temporary housing situations. For a severe disaster resulting in a request for federal assistance, local government should plan on a minimum of 3 days (72 hours) of independent operations before significant federal help can be deployed.

One of the first decisions of EMS leadership, concerning planning for mass care and sheltering, will be what type of plan to develop. If the EMS agency's role in sheltering is a supportive component of overall shelter operations, an agency standard operating procedure may suffice. If the EMS agency is responsible for managing a shelter, the agency may be tasked with developing an annex that will become part of the community's overall emergency plan. Other documents that may need to be created or revised based on the EMS role in mass care are:

- *Medical protocols.* If EMS providers are expected to dispense medications or assist shelter residents with procedures or medications not included in the normal EMS scope of practice, special protocols may need to be developed. For example, EMS providers may be asked to dispense over-the-counter medications or assist shelter occupants with allergy or insulin shots.
- *MAAs.* If EMS takes a large role in shelter operations or is required to assist at multiple shelters, planners must consider how the normal EMS call volume will be handled and whether or not to backfill stations.
- *Position descriptions.* The assignment of EMS providers to function in shelter support roles or as shelter staff may alter their normal report-to-work location, work hours, break and meal schedule, supervisory assignment, or chain of command. The agency's human resources specialists should be consulted to determine what, if any modifications must be made to employee position descriptions.
- *Organized labor agreements.* If EMS providers are represented by a labor organization (or union), the possibilities above under the "Position descriptions" heading most likely constitute a change in working conditions. Changes or additions to the EMS provider's mission or expectations, or to the providers' position description will need to be negotiated with the union prior to implementation. A labor relations specialist with the agency's human resources department should be consulted.

Whatever form the plan takes, the primary objectives of the plan should be to delineate the responsibilities and tasks of EMS personnel responsible for shelter operations, and to establish lines of authority and coordination as follows:

1. Define the roles and responsibilities of the EMS agency in support of shelter operations.
2. Identify the equipment, supplies, personnel, and other resources needed to support the operation.
3. Establish guidelines for the EMS response during disaster and shelter operations.

## Planning Considerations

Specific planning considerations will vary based on local resources, the sizes of shelters and number of occupants, and the EMS agency's specific function and level of responsibility within the shelter. The following are planning considerations that should be analyzed and implemented in the agency's shelter plan.

### Deployment Model

What is expected of the EMS agency? The level of involvement and responsibility expected of the agency, how and when it is ordered to deploy, and its mission or "scope of practice" should be clearly articulated in the written shelter procedure. Deployment models for medical support in shelters should be agreed upon in advance by the shelter management team, EMS agency, and emergency manager. Large temporary shelters such as the Houston Astrodome will have greater staffing and resource needs than a neighborhood shelter with a maximum occupancy of 40 persons. The following are some typical deployment models for EMS services in shelter operations:

- *9-1-1 point-of-service only.* The EMS agency has no specific responsibilities at shelters other than being aware of their locations and responding to medical emergencies when summoned by shelter staff.
- *Triage and intake.* One or more EMS personnel participate in the shelter's intake process to identify residents that should be segregated for medical reasons or referred to definitive care outside the shelter.
- *First aid and basic primary care—small shelter.* One or more EMS personnel provide basic primary care to shelter occupants, working independently and utilizing medical control by radio or protocol. They may assist residents by storing refrigerated medications and assisting with allergy and insulin shots, dispense over-the-counter medications, perform patient assessment, and refer seriously ill residents for definitive care outside the shelter.
- *First aid and basic primary care—medium shelter.* EMS performs duties as above for a small shelter but works with qualified shelter nurses or public health nurses.
- *First aid and basic primary care—large shelter.* In a large conference center, arena, or other facility with many hundreds or thousands of occupants, EMS personnel may provide more of a traditional EMS response role utilizing electric golf carts, bicycles, or other vehicles to respond to medical emergencies and transport patients to the shelter's medical treatment area. EMS personnel may be tasked with providing roving patrols

---

**Preplanning Practices**

Cooperative planning helps prepare the community for cooperation during an emergency. Disaster services planning (including shelter operations) should include all government organizations, NGOs, and private sector organizations with a role in an emergency, including the local emergency planning committee (LEPC), emergency management staff, and regional emergency management associations (EMAs), municipal executives, planning district commissions, not-for-profit disaster relief agencies, EMS, and public health authorities.

to interact with occupants or serve as technicians in the treatment area working with nurses, physicians, and other providers.

- *Transportation only.* EMS is responsible for staging ambulances at various shelters to transport patients to area hospitals or other locations. EMS also assists in large-scale evacuations of nonambulatory members of the community to shelters or medical facilities outside the immediate disaster area.

## Case Study

Hurricane Katrina, a category 4 storm, blew into the US Gulf Coast on Monday August 29, 2005. Homes and businesses were ruined, and huge swaths of historic New Orleans flooded as levees were overrun by the storm surge and broke apart. Hundreds of thousands of residents were displaced.

In nearby Texas, Harris County and the City of Houston immediately offered assistance and implemented shelter procedures, activating plans to open the Houston Astrodome/Reliant Center Complex as an evacuation shelter. On August 31, local government, public health services, the Harris County Hospital District, and area medical community began planning for the delivery of medical care, social services, and housing for Katrina refugees who were already on the way to Houston. More than 27,000 evacuees would eventually receive services.

On September 1, 2005, the Katrina Clinic was constructed within Reliant Arena using existing conference display materials. Over the 2-week period that the Katrina Clinic was open, more than 11,000 patients were seen. The location of the Astrodome/Reliant Center complex near the Texas College of Medicine and Baylor Medical College provided access to medical resources and providers. Medical center staff, medical students, employees from other Hospital District facilities, and volunteers from other medical practices in the community set up ambulatory care, pediatrics, physical medicine, radiology, geriatrics, mental health, and obstetrics/gynecology (OB/GYN) services within the clinic.

Fifty-six percent of evacuees seen in the clinic were age 65 or older. Evacuees were reported to be disoriented, dehydrated, emotionally distressed, and frightened. In this population, vision and hearing impairment, dementia, and other conditions contributed to many special medical needs not being immediately identified.

Services for chronic conditions were provided, including transportation for dialysis and methadone clinic treatment. The most common problem treated at Katrina Clinic was uncontrolled hypertension. Thirty-seven Katrina evacuee deaths were reported during the period the clinic operated; 23 of the deaths were in persons age 65 years or older.

An outbreak of norovirus-related acute gastroenteritis resulted in 1,000 evacuees being treated in the clinic and isolated until no longer infectious; many staff members and volunteers also became ill. Immunizations for hepatitis A, tetanus, and other illnesses were provided to more than 4,000 evacuees and 488 FEMA workers.

A National Incident Management System (NIMS)-compliant unified command was set up, with Harris County Public Health and Environmental Services (HCPHES) as the lead agency for the medical branch. Effective personnel management of the hundreds of medical volunteers was instrumental in maintaining a high standard of care; a system of credentialing for providers was implemented immediately. Doctors and nurses with expired or suspended licenses, one poseur claiming to be a doctor, and providers who attempted to set up unauthorized practices within the Astrodome were identified and removed during the time the clinic was open.

"Hurricane Katrina: Medical Response at the Houston Astrodome/Reliant Center Complex," published in *Southern Medical Journal*, provides the following lessons learned from Katrina Clinic's operation:

- Provide early screening for critical conditions such as pediatric dehydration and delirium in the elderly, with prompt referral to an emergency department.
- Case management and coordination of care must be provided for special populations including isolated elderly and disabled individuals, patients with cognitive and psychiatric disorders, diabetics, cancer

---

## Case Study, continued

patients, residents relocated from nursing homes, patients in need of dialysis, and patients with behavioral and substance abuse disorders.

● A system of credentialing medical volunteers is essential. In order to provide medical care at a shelter, providers must show proof of their level of expertise, such as a license card from a state licensing board, or a photo ID from their employer documenting their title. If a provider does not have some sort of identification, another documented provider may vouch for the undocumented provider.

● Emergency and shelter plan development should include public health officials to address sanitation, hygiene, and environmental issues in the plans.

● Tracking of residents who leave the shelter is critical for general welfare and family reunifications, particularly children, the elderly, and the disabled.

---

## Personnel

How will the agency select personnel to be assigned to work in shelter operations? In communities that utilize EMS workers as part of the shelter staff, the agency should consider formal training for EMS personnel who would receive this assignment. The American Red Cross offers several courses on shelter operations.

---

### American Red Cross Shelter Training

The following are among many courses offered by the American Red Cross available to training volunteers in the many aspects of disaster services. Many communities utilize the following four courses as the minimum training set for shelter volunteers:

● *Introduction to disaster*. Minimum training required for American Red Cross Disaster Services volunteers. Familiarizes participants with how the American Red Cross provides disaster services and provides an introduction to the various volunteer functions required during disasters.

● *Mass-care overview*. Provides an overview of mass-care activities and functions in support of disaster relief operations. Participants learn to describe the role of mass-care workers, explain how quality mass-care services are delivered, and match their interests and abilities with those needed by the American Red Cross mass-care group.

● *Shelter operations*. Prepares participants to effectively manage a shelter operations team. Includes shelter opening, operating, and closing procedures. Addresses working as a team to provide quality shelter services and common problems that occur in shelters.

● *Shelter workshop/shelter simulation*. Provides participants the opportunity to practice and demonstrate the knowledge and abilities needed to run a successful shelter operation.

---

How will the agency provide staff for shelter positions while maintaining normal response capability? An important component of the EMS agency's shelter procedure is to determine who is authorized to approve overtime for shelter operations. The plan should also address how employees are selected once overtime is authorized. This will depend on the current staffing and capability level of the agency's normal EMS response service, level of service (advanced life support or basic life support) to be provided at the shelter(s), number of personnel who have received shelter training, existing agency hire-back (equitable overtime rotation) procedures, and the availability of volunteers.

EMS agencies that may have to utilize employee recalls to support staffing for disaster or other operations should designate members subject to emergency, forced recall to work as emergency essential or mission essential employees. This designation should be included in the employee's position description so that it is enforceable. Along with emergency essential designation, the employer is responsible for making sure that employees are aware of their designation and that accurate and up-to-date recall lists are maintained. The EMS agency should also assist essential employees in making sure that they have family emergency plans and that family members are educated on what to do and where to go in a disaster, since the EMS provider may be at work.

In the event that a disaster impacts normal communications, the EMS agency should preplan what essential employees should do. Options include having employees automatically report to specific locations for instructions or to monitor specific emergency alert system (EAS) radio stations for instructions.

Since employees from multiple departments of local government as well as NGO volunteers may be placed together in a work unit and be remote from their normal duty station, a standardized tracking system should be used to roster staff and account for time. ICS Form 211 "Incident Check-In List" is an ideal format for rostering personnel from multiple agencies and departments (see **Figure 8-1**). Copies of ICS 211 and timekeeping records should be periodically forwarded to the timekeeping unit (finance section).

## Command

Command structure for shelter management will vary among localities based on the size of the emergency management infrastructure and response resources, community size, and the preferences of the emergency management staff. The command structure should be compliant with the NIMS and utilize the principles and standard terminology of the incident command system (ICS). Preplanning, both in the larger municipal emergency plan and individual agency procedures, should emphasize the chosen command organization and emphasize lines of authority.

Many community and incident-specific factors will influence exactly where shelter management operations and medical support functions are placed in the ICS structure. Planners should not focus on an ICS organizational chart and how to fill in the blanks, but instead should start with the resources that preplanning indicates will be needed and build the organizational chart around those resources. The resources should be organized into a structure with unity of command, clear lines of reporting, common sense function and communications arrangements, and a manageable span of control and supervisory structure. The following case study illustrates how to create an emergency management ICS organization based on needs identified through the preplanning process.

## Navy Region Mid-Atlantic Fire & Emergency Services

| INCIDENT CHECK-IN LIST | | | | Incident Name | | | | Check-in Location | | | | Date/Time |
|---|---|---|---|---|---|---|---|---|---|---|---|---|
| Specify type of equipment contained on this sheet or misc. | | | | | | | | | | | | |
| Agency | SR ST TF | Type | ID No. or Name | Date/ Time In | Date/ Time Out | Leader/ Supervisor | Total # Persons | Home Base | Method of Travel | Incident Assign. | Assignment Location |
| | SR ST TF | | | | | | | | | Y/N | |

**Figure 8-1** ICS Form 211, Incident Check-In List.

| | | | | | | | | | | | |
|---|---|---|---|---|---|---|---|---|---|---|---|
| | SR ST TF | | | | | | | | | Y/N | |
| | SR ST TF | | | | | | | | | Y/N | |
| | SR ST TF | | | | | | | | | Y/N | |
| | SR ST TF | | | | | | | | | Y/N | |
| | SR ST TF | | | | | | | | | Y/N | |
| | SR ST TF | | | | | | | | | Y/N | |
| | SR ST TF | | | | | | | | | Y/N | |
| | SR ST TF | | | | | | | | | Y/N | |
| | SR ST TF | | | | | | | | | Y/N | |
| | SR ST TF | | | | | | | | | Y/N | |
| | SR ST TF | | | | | | | | | Y/N | |
| | SR ST TF | | | | | | | | | Y/N | |
| | SR ST TF | | | | | | | | | Y/N | |
| Page ____ of ____ | | Prepared by (Name and position); use back for remarks | | | | | | | | Incoming personnel traveling more than 4 hours should report to REHAB for baseline vital signs, hydration, food, and rest prior to receiving an assignment. | |

**Figure 8-1** ICS Form 211, Incident Check-In List.
Courtesy of Navy Region Mid Atlantic Fire & Emergency Services.

## Case Study

### Monroe County

4,928 total square miles

*County government*: Elected board of supervisors, full-time county manager.

County (unincorporated area) contains 45,000 citizens.

*continues*

## Case Study, continued

Monroe Township is the county seat, containing 27,000 citizens in 84 square miles.

*Town government*: Elected mayor and town council, full-time town manager

*Emergency management staff*: The county employs a full-time emergency manager (EM); Monroe Township's police chief serves as the town's EM.

*Public safety*—The Monroe County sheriff's department performs law enforcement, investigation, and patrol services with jurisdiction over the entire county. A total of 77 deputies and investigators also provide courthouse security and run the county jail. The sheriff is elected. Monroe Township's police department provides law enforcement to the incorporated township with 10 sworn officers, including the police chief. State police patrol the four-lane US highway that bisects the county; there are normally no more than two troopers on duty at any one time.

*Emergency services*—Monroe County emergency services employs a full-time emergency services director, fire marshal, training and grants coordinator with the rank of lieutenant, and brigade chief (who functions as the daytime battalion chief for fire and EMS and as the daytime volunteer coordinator). All of the above staff work Monday through Friday from 8 am to 4 pm. Fire, police, and EMS dispatch is performed by the sheriff's department.

The county has three paid EMS supervisors with the rank of captain that rotate 24-hour shifts so that one supervisor is always on duty. The county staffs three, one-person, paramedic-level quick response vehicles Monday through Friday from 6 am to 5 pm. These three paramedic units are posted throughout the county at strategic locations based on call volume.

Ambulance service is provided by seven independent volunteer rescue squads. One private, hospital-based ambulance service also operates in the county, primarily providing interfacility transports. The private service picks up 9-1-1 calls occasionally when it has a unit available by MAA.

Fire protection is provided by a total of nine all-volunteer fire departments including the township's department, which has two stations (total of 10 stations in the county). Monroe Township has two paid firefighters who act as driver-operators during the daytime hours to supplement the volunteers at its two stations. The volunteer department chiefs and deputy chiefs rotate as the night time brigade chief for the county.

*Hospitals*—The county has one hospital. Monroe Memorial is a 60-bed community hospital. It has a six-bed labor and delivery unit, six-bed medical-surgical intensive care unit, six-bed medical-surgical step-down unit, 10-bed in-patient psychiatric unit, and 14-bed emergency room. The hospital has a CT scanner, and two noninterventional cardiologists; patients who need stroke care or cardiac catheterization are transported to a larger city medical center 35 miles away. The city medical center is also the closest trauma center.

The county Emergency Management Committee meets quarterly. It is comprised of the county EM, Monroe Township's police chief and public works director, the county health department's director and epidemiologist, the county public works and emergency services directors, the county's paid emergency services brigade chief, the Red Cross chapter director, an under sheriff and emergency communications center supervisor from the sheriff's department, nursing director and security chief from Monroe Memorial Hospital, and a state police division officer. Administrative support for the committee is provided by a secretary from the county manager's office. The Emergency Management Committee has joint meetings with the Local Emergency Planning Committee (LEPC) twice per year.

*Scenario*: Hurricane season is approaching, and the county's EM has just returned from the national hurricane conference and attended several sessions on population sheltering. The county has become NIMS-compliant within the past 2 years. The county EM suggests reworking the command structure because of some perceived disorganization and after action report comments from the last major hurricane that the county experienced.

When Hurricane Zelda struck the county in August 2 years ago, there was significant residential and commercial roof damage, rendering 300 properties temporarily uninhabitable. The high winds also caused widespread power outages. It took the electricity cooperative 12 days to fully restore power to 80% of the county; it took an additional 10 days to restore power to all customers in the most rural parts of the county.

Three shelters were opened, two in Monroe Township and one in the northern part of the county. Residents trickled into the shelters during the first 24 hours, and the decision was made to close one of the Township shelters. After the fourth day with no power, the two remaining shelters were flooded with residents seeking assistance and respite from the heat, including a large percentage of elderly residents. 9-1-1 calls to county emergency services spiked as residents with chronic illness had no electricity to power home oxygen generation units, nebulizer pumps, and other equipment. Fire department units, state department of transportation workers, and county public works staff were directed to cut trees to open roads in areas where patients with urgent dialysis and other medical needs were located because their normal caregivers and private ambulance transport services had been unable to reach their homes.

9-1-1 calls for EMS assistance at the shelters spiked on days 4 through 6 as elderly and ill patients began to run out of medications used to manage chronic illness. Due to landline phone outages and many local doctor's offices and clinics being closed due to power outages, shelter staff began calling 9-1-1 for ambulance transport service for the patients in need of dialysis and other routine care that were being brought to the shelters. Volunteer EMS workers began self-dispatching themselves back to the shelters to pick up other patients they had noticed while they had picked up their previous transport. After day 6, local businesses began to reopen as power was reestablished, and the number of available EMS volunteers began to dwindle; dispatchers began "stacking" calls. Call volume began tapering off on day 7 as power was restored to more areas, many roads were cleared, and shelter residents began being able to return to their own residences or stayed with family members.

The EM committee also analyzed the command structure used during Hurricane Zelda. During the hurricane, shelter operations were organized by the human services unit (services branch, logistics section) in the command organization. Human services also includes behavioral health and social services and the community service board (the county's mental health service). The committee came to the conclusion that Monroe county's human services organizations' staffs were too small to adequately organize and operate the shelter command elements in addition to the extensive social work and case management tasks that had to be performed during the hurricane—shelter operations and all of the other functions performed by human services exceeded the span of control of the small number of human service managers. Furthermore, the committee thought that human services managers were ill-equipped to effectively deal with agencies more accustomed to act as "responders."

Based on issues identified during the analysis of the Zelda response, the EM committee made the following changes to the county's incident command organization and response plan:

- Shelter operations were moved to their own branch in the operations section. An experienced county emergency services staff member will lead the branch, which will include American Red Cross shelter teams, a medical support unit, and a transportation unit.
- A transportation unit was created within the shelter branch. The unit will be staffed by volunteer EMS workers and private ambulance companies. The county will create a contract for private ambulance company support that can be executed when multiple shelters are opened. The shelter's transportation unit resources will be separate from the normal 9-1-1 EMS assets and will be controlled by the shelter branch director.
- A medical support unit was created within the shelter branch. This unit will be made up of public health nurses and volunteer EMS providers. Medical support teams will be assigned to each shelter and will communicate with the medical unit leader for coordinated and centralized medical control and transportation requests.

● Efficient use of state resources such as ambulance task forces and statewide mutual aid will be made through EOC requests.

The incident command organizational chart for the case study is intended for illustrative purposes only; local resources and incident management structure may result in a different organization (see **Figure 8-2**).

As in the previous case study, planning activities should be coordinated among the various government and nongovernment agencies that will be part of the response. Interaction through coordinated planning sessions and exercises will introduce and reinforce ICS concepts to organizations that do not routinely work in "response mode." The utilization of NIMS terminology, practices, and forms during routine agency operations further assists with familiarity with NIMS and ICS principles, and prepares agencies to utilize these concepts and practices in an emergency.

## Supply and Logistics

Shelters require significant supplies and equipment. The basics are cots, bedding, and sanitation supplies. Many shelters also provide preassembled personal comfort hygiene kits. These supplies may be cached in a storage area on the shelter property, warehoused in bulk in a separate location, or stored in trailers or shipping containers that would need to be transported to each shelter. Basic medical supplies for first aid and primary care should be assembled and pre-staged by the agency responsible for medical support. The supply component is often easier than the logistics component: Logistics entails maintaining the equipment in serviceable condition, replacing supplies that fall outside their shelf life, and moving the cache to where it is needed.

Funding for shelter medical supplies may be supported by the municipal emergency management organization, the American Red Cross, or another shelter coordinating agency. Keeping thorough records during shelter operations is important for potential reimbursement for supplies used in an emergency.

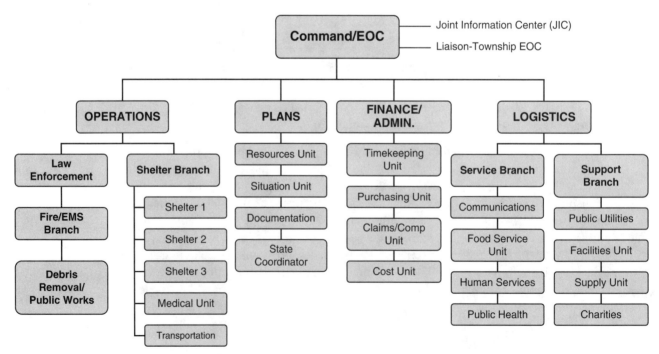

**Figure 8-2** Monroe County Hurricane Recovery/Emergency Shelter Organizational Chart.

If the EMS agency is required to absorb the cost of shelter caches out of its normal operating budget, consider building the cache in modules so that at least part of the shelter cache may also be used for other purposes like first aid and standby operations at large public events or mass-casualty operations. Area hotels and motels may donate towels and other linens that they no longer consider serviceable for guest use.

The shelter manager will likely have a kit with administrative supplies, signs, forms used for screening and check-in, and templates for reports. The leader of each shelter medical support unit should also have a kit that includes the forms to be used for patient care record keeping, plastic baggies and labels for storing and labeling patient medications, and the forms needed for situation reports and personnel accountability.

## Public Affairs

Shelter staff should be briefed on the municipality's public affairs plan and procedures. Normally, all media inquiries should be directed to the incident's designated public affairs officer or joint information center (JIC). Because shelters will be remote from the emergency operations center, media outlets will approach shelter staff for information and comments. A procedure to address these approaches should be developed and briefed to all shelter staff. Some agencies allow shelter staff to be interviewed by the media contingent on (1) the shelter manager's approval and (2) that the staffer may only discuss his or her particular role in operations. Whatever the policy, it should be planned in advance and be available at each shelter in the operations plan or as part of the shelter manager's kit.

# Creating a Medical Needs Shelter

Special needs patients are those that require ongoing care or supervision, and who are dependent on family members, home health providers, or other medical professionals for medical care and support with activities of daily living. Many special needs patients live at home and depend on family and visits from home health nurses, therapists, and other caregivers. Others are residents of nursing homes or other licensed care facilities. Special needs patients may have mobility restrictions, chronic illnesses, or are recovering from strokes, fractures, or other medical conditions. This category may include terminally ill persons receiving hospice care. Typical conditions requiring medical support are patients that use home oxygen, with dialysis requirements, or with diabetes management requirements. This category of residents is generally not sick enough to be in the hospital, but require some type of ongoing care.

When multiple shelters are opened within a jurisdiction, it is reasonable to expect a few residents with special medical needs to show up at most shelters; a significant number of residents will require prescription medication refills during their time at the shelter. If the jurisdiction provides only minimal medical support staff and resources for each shelter, it may consolidate these residents at one or more medical needs shelters. When patients with special medical needs are screened as part of the check-in process at regular shelters, they can be identified and transported with their family members or caregivers to the medical needs shelter. Licensed care facilities such as nursing, rehabilitative, or group homes may also make a local special needs shelter their shelter of last resort.

## EMS Preplanning and Public Education for Special Needs Persons

The mission of disaster education and planning should be coordinated by the jurisdiction's emergency management program, and may include the Red Cross and other NGOs, as well as fire and EMS agencies. EMS agencies will play a large role in any mass evacuation of special needs persons; even if EMS does not have a role in managing shelters, it will likely be extensively involved in transporting patients. Therefore, EMS should be proactive in public education activities that will help special needs persons and licensed care facilities maintain the patients' continuity and level of care.

The focus of public education should be on the caregiver's role in planning for the continuity of care for the patient during a disaster. This responsibility includes planning for the possibility of sheltering in place, being evacuated, and temporary placement in a disaster shelter (either a regular shelter or medical needs shelter). Area senior organizations and emergency management staff can collaborate on the development of educational materials on how to prepare for disasters. Lists of important items to prepare in a "go bag" for evacuation are also valuable (see **Table 8-2**). EMS can assist by providing these educational materials to special needs patients it encounters during normal operations, at public events like health fairs, at neighborhood and civic league presentations, and during preplanning visits to nursing homes and other licensed care facilities. Special needs patients should also be encouraged to maintain an updated emergency information form (EIF) that identifies their medical history, conditions, and medications.

Licensed care facilities are also responsible for preparing their facilities and staffs for operations during disasters. Ideally, these facilities will have evacuation plans and transportation resources that relocate their populations to like facilities in areas unaffected by the disaster or discharge patients to family members. It is very important that staff members be aware of the need for caregivers to accompany their patients to the shelter and stay with them in the shelter to provide care. Licensed care facility staff members, like emergency services employees, should have family emergency plans that prepare their families for the likelihood that they will remain at work during a disaster.

Home health care agencies should maintain communication with emergency management officials and maintain lists of high-risk clients and those with significant mobility challenges; EMS can help in this area by actively interacting with home health care providers. Knowledge of high-risk patients could also be an asset for normal EMS response preplanning.

## Planning Objectives

The objectives in planning for a special needs shelter are very similar to those for a normal shelter, but with a focus on medical and emergency shelter needs of special needs persons. The plan should address activities to be performed before, during, and after a disaster.

1. Define the roles and responsibilities of government agencies and community organizations involved with the care and sheltering of special needs persons.
2. Identify the facilities and infrastructure needed to provide shelter for special needs persons.
3. Identify the resources needed to operate a medical needs shelter.
4. Establish guidelines for disaster response to special needs persons and operations and staffing of medical needs shelters.

## Community Planning and Education Goals

The following goals rely heavily on multidisciplinary preplanning and coordination as well as effective public education activities for their validity in a particular jurisdiction.

- Special needs persons who live independently are encouraged to have their own support network and to preidentify an evacuation site (friends, family, hotel) outside the area if evacuation becomes necessary.
- Special needs persons should be prepared to be self-sufficient in their homes with limited support for up to 72 hours.
- Licensed care facilities should be prepared to meet the medical needs of their staff and residents in emergencies.

**Table 8-2** Emergency Supplies Checklist

In case of a serious disaster, relief workers will be on the scene, but they cannot reach everyone immediately. Help could come in hours, or it may take days. To be prepared, everyone should be able to cope with the emergency until help arrives. One way to prepare is to assemble a disaster supplies kit. Once a disaster hits, there will not be time to shop or search for supplies. Following a serious disaster, it is important to remember that there may be no electricity, gas, water, or telephone service. EMS should plan for enough supplies to last at least 3 days.

**Necessities:**
- *Several flashlights.* By the bed and around the house; electricity may be out
- *Battery-operated radio.* To listen for information about the emergency
- *Extra batteries.* For flashlight, radio, hearing aide, or other medical devices
- *Bottled water for 3 days.* 3 gallons per person
- *Nonperishable, ready-to-eat food for 3 days.* Dried fruit, canned tuna, stew, beans, canned fruit juices, nuts, crackers, etc
- *Manual can opener.* To open canned food
- *First aid kit.* Include a first aid handbook, gauze, bandages, scissors, tape, disinfectants, antiseptics, aspirin, and other over-the-counter medications
- *Extra prescription medication to last for 5 days.* And a copy of the prescriptions
- *Plastic garbage bags and duct tape.* For personal waste and quick repairs
- *Emergency health information card.* Include a copy in the disaster supplies kit
- *Whistle or loud bell.* To attract attention if trapped
- *Adjustable wrench.* For gas and water shutoff

**Other important items:**
- *Extra eyeglasses or hearing aid.* Original equipment may become lost or misplaced
- *Extra walking aids.* Equipment may be damaged; powered equipment may not be able to be recharged without electricity
- *Extra set of keys.* In case the original set cannot be accessed
- *Pet food and extra water for pets.*
- *Shoes under the bed.* To protect feet from broken glass from picture frames, lamps, etc
- *Money.* Banks may be closed, plus quarters for pay phones, vending machines
- *Copies of key documents.* Will, insurance policies, credit cards, and bank accounts, etc
- *Blankets.* To keep warm if heat is unavailable for an extended period

**Emergency "Go Kit":**
- *Prepare an emergency "Go Kit"* that could be grabbed and taken if there is a need to evacuate. Along with a change of clothes, include necessary medications, personal hygiene supplies, any special sanitary aids, and important contact information or telephone numbers. Store these items in an easy-to-carry container such as a backpack or duffel bag.

Courtesy of Alameda County Operational Area Emergency Management Organization, Alameda County, CA.

- Licensed care facilities should develop and exercise workable evacuation and transportation plans and be capable of relocating their patients to like facilities in areas unaffected by the disaster.

## Assumptions

No matter the level of preparedness, there will be special needs persons who:

- Suffer an exacerbation of their medical condition or otherwise deteriorate
- Experience a mechanical failure of a home medical device

- Do not have generators to power home medical devices
- Have their care interrupted due to a primary caregiver being affected by the disaster

Likewise, either because of a lack of planning or situations caused by the disaster, there will be licensed care facilities that have problems executing the facility care or evacuation plan resulting in their resident population needing care and shelter.

## Activation

The emergency management team will have several variables to consider in deciding whether to activate medical needs shelters. Case management support staff in normal shelters may be able to place special needs patients with family members or hotels outside the disaster area. Some patients with exacerbations in their conditions may need to be hospitalized. Shelter staff will be making periodic reports on their occupancy to the shelter branch manager or EOC. Based on the number of special needs persons checking into regular shelters and any problems in evacuating local licensed care facilities, the decision may be made to activate one or more medical needs shelters.

Family members or other caregivers should accompany the patient to the medical needs shelter. Licensed care facilities who evacuate patients to medical needs shelters should bring adequate staff, including nursing support (when required), and medical records for their residents. Family and home health providers and licensed care facilities should bring enough supplies, medications, oxygen, and equipment to care for their patients for a minimum of 72 hours. Care providers who relocate to the medical needs shelter with their patients should have the responsibility for providing routine care and administering medications.

## Supplies, Support, and Logistics

Patients with special medical needs are likely to require use of medical equipment such as infusion pumps, nebulizer pumps, and other devices that will increase the need for electrical outlets in medical needs shelters compared to normal emergency shelters. Plan for a facilities technician or electrician to be part of the initial setup staff so that extension cords and junction boxes can be configured safely. Overloading electrical outlets and using extension cords with insufficient ratings can be a fire hazard. It is also possible for demand to exceed the supply of electricity, particularly when generator power is being used.

While caregivers should plan on bringing supplies, medications, and equipment to last their patient for 3 days, there will be patients who arrive at the shelter without the needed supplies for a variety of reasons. Some arrivals will be impoverished, will have had to make a quick escape, or were just unprepared. Planning for a medical needs shelter should include a cache of basic supplies for medical care, hygiene, and sanitation. Additionally, just as the shelter manager has a kit that includes signs and registration forms, the medical providers need a kit that includes patient care forms, identification bracelets, and baggies and labels for medications. **Table 8-3** describes the recommended medical supply cache inventory for a medical needs shelter.

The shelter operations plan must include a plan for moving the cache from storage to where it is needed. Once built and inventoried, the medical needs shelter cache should be programmed for periodic checks and testing just like any other EMS equipment, including maintaining the supplies within their shelf life and testing and maintenance of medical equipment.

Shelter support volunteers at a medical needs shelter will spend more time with sanitation and hygiene tasks than their counterparts at normal emergency shelters. Many of the residents of a medical needs shelter may need bedpans and urinals for their toileting, or use incontinent supplies like adult diapers and absorbent pads. An area for storage and disposal of used hygiene and toileting supplies should be planned and designated in advance with sanitation of the shelter and odor control in mind.

**Table 8-3** Medical Needs Shelter Medical Supply Cache Inventory

| Quantity | Item/Description | Quantity | Item/Description |
|---|---|---|---|
| 1 bottle | Nonaspirin pain reliever, 100/bottle | 2 dozen | Applicators, cotton-tipped |
| 2 bottles | Nonaspirin pain reliever, pediatric, liquid | 50 | Tongue depressors, sterile |
| 2 | Epi-Pen | 1 | Betadine scrub, bottle |
| 50 | Diphenhydramine capsules, 25 mg | 10 | Bed pans, disposable |
| 50 | Triple antibiotic ointment, unit dose | 10 | Urinals, disposable |
| 50 | Antipruritic ointment, unit dose | 12 | Baby bottles |
| 2 boxes | Antacid, low sodium, 25/box | 300 | Alcohol prep pads |
| 1 bottle | First aid spray or topical antiseptic | 50 | Biohazard waste bags |
| 1 bottle | Aspirin, 5 grain, 100/bottle | 3 bottles | Body lotion, moisturizing |
| 100 | Blood glucose testing strips | 3 bottles | Insect repellent |
| 1 | Glucometer | 10 | Basins, hospital-style, disposable |
| 100 | Lancets | 2 | Buckets, 3 gallon |
| 12 | Roller gauze bandages | 2 | Chlorine bleach, gallon |
| 1 | Can opener | 100 | Chux pads |
| 24 | Dressing, nonadherent, sterile, 4 × 4 | 1 box | Colostomy bags, box |
| 4 | Elastic bandages, 3-inch | 3 dozen | Diapers, newborn, medium, and large |
| 1 | Flashlight and batteries, per staff member | 3 dozen | Diapers, adult |
| 4 | Forceps or large tweezers | 10 | Emesis basin or bags, disposable |
| 4 | Scissors | 8 boxes | Facial tissues |
| 4 boxes | Gloves, nitrile small | 24 | Surgical/dust masks |
| 4 boxes | Gloves, nitrile, medium | 2 | High-efficiency particulate air (HEPA) respirator, per staff member |
| 4 boxes | Gloves, nitrile, large | 2 cases | Formula, infant, powdered |
| 4 boxes | Gloves, nitrile, X-large | 2 cases | Premoistened towelettes, 200/case |
| 4 | Sterile water for irrigation, 1-L bottle | 100 | Identification bracelets |
| 25 | Insulin syringes | 1 case | Formula, soy |

*continues*

**Table 8-3**  (Continued)

| Quantity | Item/Description | Quantity | Item/Description |
|---|---|---|---|
| 1 | Irrigation kit | 50 | Plastic ziplock baggies |
| 48 | Anti-diarrheal, unit dose tablets | 24 | Disposable cold packs |
| 4 | Oxygen, D-cylinder | 12 | Sharpie markers |
| 2 | Portable oxygen regulator | 1 case | Paper cups |
| 4 each | Oxygen mask and cannula | 1 case | Paper towels |
| 1 | Petroleum jelly | 24 | Safety pins |
| 24 | Nonpetroleum lubricant, unit dose pack | 24 | Sanitary napkins |
| 1 | Sphygmomanometer and cuff, large adult | 2 | Sharps container |
| 1 | Sphygmomanometer and cuff, adult | 10 | Alcohol-based hand cleaner foam |
| 1 | Sphygmomanometer and cuff, pediatric | 10 | Disinfectant hospital wipes, 100/tub |
| 1 | Stethoscope | 1 | Fluid spill kit |
| 1 | Thermometer | 1 | Catheter tube and bag set |
| 100 | Cots | 2 | Walkers |
| 100 | Blankets | 200 | Sheets |
| 100 | Patient belonging bags | 100 | Pillows, disposable |
| 24 | Throat lozenges, unit dose | 1 | Shelter manager kit and forms |
| | | 1 | Shelter operations plan |

*Note:* Suggested for 100 people, for 3 days.

Courtesy of Alameda County Operational Area Emergency Management Organization, Alameda County, CA.

Obtaining diabetic supplies for evacuees in the first few days after Hurricane Katrina was very problematic for emergency shelters due to availability of pharmaceuticals; some patients had evacuated without medical records and relied on memory for their medication regimen. Often the minimal diabetic supplies available at shelters did not match the patient's normal regimen. Similarly, insulin supplies in Florida were reported to be exhausted within the first 24 hours after Hurricane Andrew in 1992. EMS planners should analyze various likely shelter scenarios in an attempt to anticipate what type of pharmacy cache will be appropriate for their planned shelters. Based on the community's size and location, the local public health service may have an existing cache. Localities with municipal hospital authorities should involve hospital pharmacy directors in shelter logistics planning. For communities with no municipal hospital authority or robust public health pharmacy cache, planners should consider contracting with retail pharmacies to ensure adequate medications will be available.

## Medical Needs Shelter Staff

Ideally, patient care attendants, nursing assistants, and family caregivers will accompany each special needs patient to the shelter. It is likely that at least some patients will arrive without a caregiver. Additionally, many patient care assistants and nursing assistants may need the assistance and supervision of a nurse, particularly over a period of several days. A medical needs shelter will need all of the normal shelter staff positions, plus the following medical specialists:

- *Registered nurses.* Nurses from the public health department, American Red Cross, or other agency provide nursing care and overall medical oversight at the medical needs shelter and provide guidance to nonlicensed medical support personnel such as nursing assistants.
- *Paramedics.* Provide acute care, administer medications, and troubleshoot problems with medical equipment and oxygen delivery.
- *Case managers.* Social services or American Red Cross case managers help in coordinating care, arranging for placement of patients in facilities outside of the disaster area, arrange for prescription refills, and ensure necessary ongoing specialty care like dialysis is provided.

The number of staff members required will be dictated by the staff-to-patient ratio decided in advance by shelter planners and emergency management, population size of the shelter, compliance with instructions for caregivers to come with the patients, acuity level of the patients, and shift schedules and length.

## Records and Reports

Accurate written records are essential for all shelter operations for reimbursement purposes. It is also very important to track patients as they are moved within the shelter, within the shelter system, and as they are discharged to family or placed in other care facilities. The American Red Cross normally provides welfare tracking during disasters so that families can be reunited. While each municipality will develop its own record keeping system, the following are some written reports typical of all shelter operations:

### Employee/Volunteer Records

As discussed earlier in the chapter, personnel record keeping is essential for eventual reimbursement from the state or federal government for operational costs, particularly overtime. It is also necessary to be able to verify any volunteer or employee's claim for overtime or injury compensation. The employee's assignments during the disaster, the date and place assigned and specific function, release date, days and hours worked, and any travel costs should be recorded. The ICS 211 form is ideal for keeping records of personnel from multiple agencies who are assigned to work together as a unit. Daily or shift time sheets should also be kept. Timekeeping and ICS 211 forms should be periodically forwarded to the timekeeping unit in the finance section.

### Supply and Equipment Costs

While the emergency management organization's purchasing unit (finance section) may facilitate large purchases and award contracts on behalf of the municipality, there are many smaller costs that must be tracked at the unit or branch level. NGOs such as the American Red Cross or Salvation Army should track funds expended on supplies and feeding operations. Individual shelters or units may be issued petty cash or credit cards for small purchases; these purchases should be categorized and tracked. Costs of any rental equipment, fuel for generators, the cost of vouchers for prescriptions, and other incidental costs should be recorded.

### Shelter Status Report

Depending on the incident and how quickly conditions change, the shelter status report may be required daily or several times a day. This is a basic status report that provides information on the number of shelter occupants, number of beds available, a list of resources needed and in what quantity, and a brief report of any problems or incidents.

### Transportation Log

This is a record of all transports performed by the transportation unit. The purpose of the log is to track patients as they are moved from shelters to other shelters, hospitals, or are discharged or placed in other care facilities.

### After Action Report

After every incident, an AAR should be prepared by each unit and submitted to the branch director. The report includes response actions taken, issues that were identified, and recommendations for corrective actions. Topics may include adequacy of supplies and personnel, security issues, incidents, training needs, and communications issues.

## Decedent Affairs

Unfortunately when a jurisdiction is operating multiple shelters, including medical needs shelters over several days, it is likely that one or more of the shelters may experience a death. Whether due to completely natural causes or a medical condition aggravated by the conditions of the disaster, preplanning is essential for this situation to be handled in a professional and calm manner. Consider the following when incorporating decedent affairs into the agency procedure or local emergency plan:

- Designate an area in each shelter, in advance, for temporary storage of remains.
- Negotiate contracts in advance with local funeral directors that can be executed in the event of a decedent with no family members or next of kin that can be contacted.
- Incorporate a clear reporting process into the agency's procedure/plan.
- Identify the proper reporting contacts for death investigations in advance (police, medical examiner, etc) based on local laws and protocols.
- Determine in advance who is authorized to release information to the public and the media about the deceased.

## Demobilization

Medical needs shelters are temporary accommodations operated only as long as is necessary to place residents in more appropriate facilities. As the situation in the surrounding community improves, shelter managers should plan for special needs patients to be transferred out of the shelter according to the following priorities:

1. Discharge patients to their home or original licensed care facility.
2. For patients whose homes are damaged or inaccessible, discharge patients who normally live independently to the care of family, friends, or another willing caregiver.
3. Transfer patients to a facility similar to their original licensed care facility that has the capacity to accept them.
4. As patient populations dwindle, consolidate medical needs shelters and close those that are no longer necessary.
5. If the community has profound damage with a long recovery period expected, transfer the remaining patients to family members or licensed care facilities outside the disaster area.

Shelter cache supplies should be inventoried and equipment cleaned, disinfected, and repacked. All documents and records should be turned over to the shelter branch manager. Employees should be solicited for AAR feedback prior to being released to their home agency.

EMS agencies must be aware of where they fit in the local disaster plan (including sheltering), and establish internal plans detailing the specifics of how they will carry out the expected roles.

## Incorporating Shelters into Preplans

Many types of natural and man-made disasters may result in the need for communities to provide temporary, mass-care shelters for displaced residents; EMS agencies may be tasked with providing varying levels of support in the sheltering process. An important aspect of planning for shelter operations is the method that the agency will use to document its efforts, time, and expenses, since state and federal disaster financial support may be available to reimburse local disaster relief partners. MAAs are important planning tools because they specify in advance the type and level of support between entities and establish reimbursement methods, legal liability, and responsibility for workers' compensation in advance.

The NRF emphasizes cooperative and engaged partnerships among government and NGOs, planning for a tiered response that is flexible and adapts to the type of response required, the readiness to act when needed, and an organized system of unified command. Planning activities should include all agencies and partners anticipated to be involved in the response. The daily, routine use of ICS processes and forms during nondisaster operations is likely to improve familiarity with the command system and improve interagency function and cooperation during a real emergency.

The EMS agency may need to create or revise a number of plans and documents as it prepares to support shelter operations, including medical protocols for primary care, employee position descriptions, and standard operating procedures. The command structure to be utilized for shelter operations should be planned in advance. The command structure should be compliant with NIMS, must be capable of efficient supervision and accountability of staff, and must mesh into the locality's overall emergency management command system.

The EMS agency can play a valuable role in assisting individual members of the community with specific medical needs and licensed care facilities in planning for continuity of care during emergencies. Public events and facility preplanning visits are good opportunities to provide information on how to prepare for evacuation and what residents and caregivers should bring to temporary shelters. Licensed care facilities should be encouraged to develop their own emergency plans and to prepare caregivers for the need to accompany their patients and remain with them at mass-care shelters.

## Selected References

Alameda County Operational Area Emergency Management Organization. *Alameda County Disaster Shelter Plan for Medically Fragile Persons.* Alameda, CA: Alameda County Operational Area Emergency Management Organization; 2004.

Alson, R, Alexander, D, et al.: Analysis of medical treatment at a field hospital following Hurricane Andrew. *Ann Emerg Med* 1992;22:1721–1728.

American Red Cross. *Introduction to Disaster Services Fact Sheet,* DSGEN201C; 2006.

American Red Cross. *Mass Care Overview Fact Sheet,* DSMCC200A; 2007.

American Red Cross. *Shelter Operations Fact Sheet,* ARC3068-11; 2006.

American Red Cross. *Shelter Simulation Fact Sheet,* ARC3068-12; 2006.

Centers for Disease Control and Prevention: *Chemical Agents: Facts Sheltering in place.* US Department of Health and Human Services; August 16, 2006.

Congressional Charter of the American National Red Cross: *36 USC;* May, 2007.

*Disaster Relief,* U.S. Code Title 42, chapter 68.

Fernandez, LS, Byard, D, et al.: Frail elderly as disaster victims: Emergency management strategies. *Prehosp Disaster Med* 2002;17(2):67–74.

Gavagan, TF, Smart, K, et al.: Hurricane Katrina: Medical response at the Houston Astrodome/Reliant Center Complex. *South Med J* 2006;99(9):933–939.

Howe, E, Victor, D, et al.: Chief complaints, diagnoses, and medications prescribed seven weeks post-Katrina in New Orleans. *Prehosp Disaster Med* 2008;23(1):41–47.

Laditka, SB, Laditka, JN, et al.: Disaster preparedness for vulnerable persons receiving in-home, long-term care in South Carolina. *Prehosp Disaster Med* 2008;23(2):133–142.

Landesman, LY: *Public Health Management of Disasters: The Practice Guide.* 2nd ed. Washington, D.C.: American Public Health Association; 2005.

Miller, AC and Arquilla, B: Chronic diseases and natural hazards: Impact of disasters on diabetic, renal, and cardiac patients. *Prehosp Disaster Med* 2008;23(3):185–194.

National Association of Emergency Managers: *Emergency Management Assistance Compact Overview.* Lexington, KY. http://www.nemaweb.org. Accessed December 1, 2009.

State of California. *California Emergency Services Act*, definition, section 8558(a).

United States Department of Homeland Security: *National Response Framework;* January 2008. http://www.dhs.gov/files/programs/editorial_0566.shtm. Accessed December 1, 2009.

United States Department of Homeland Security: Shelter operations: Establishing a quiet room to calm residents with mental illness. *Lessons Learned Information Sharing.* https://www.llis.dhs.gov/index.do.

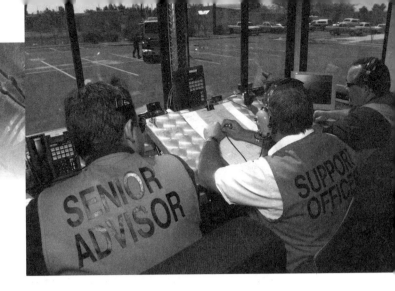

# Chapter 9

# Coordination

## Why Coordinate?

Emergency response agencies tend to coordinate with outside organizations only when needed. Many emergency medical services (EMS) agencies feel that interagency coordination is done on scene or as an incident develops, rather than something to be done ahead of time, because they view their agencies as response-only and not preplanning-type agencies. Those agencies that have dealt with large incidents know that this is not the case.

Several after action reports (AARs) and critiques of major incidents have shown that response without coordination leads to several negative results (see **Figure 9-1**). One result is increased suffering on the part of patients, the public, and responders. This human suffering is a result of missed actions, wasting of resources, or duplication of effort by responding agencies. Three major examples of the results of a lack of coordination are the September 11, 2001 attack in New York City, as well as response failures during Hurricanes Katrina and Rita. These experiences show that certain agencies will take it upon themselves to respond to an incident without adequate coordination. These agencies, although they provide valuable resources, can potentially block other resources that are specifically needed from getting in. The agencies utilize resources to take care of their responders that may have been used to direct the operations of other agencies incorporated into the response plan, and they create problems by overloading the system and hindering the ability of the incident command system (ICS) and the incident commanders on scene to direct and use these newly arrived responders efficiently.

### "The Five Ps"

EMS agencies may refer to "the five Ps" to motivate the incorporation of coordination into event or incident preplans: "Prior Planning Prevents Poor Performance." Very simply, prior planning prevents response agencies from wasting resources that are not needed. A well-planned, coordinated response by multiple agencies will be more efficient and will decrease human suffering. Consider the following case study:

## Case Study

Prior planning was evident during the response to Hurricane Ike, which hit on September 12, 2008. After learning from mistakes made during Hurricane Katrina, American Medical Response (AMR) built a cadre of

*continues*

---

**Case Study, continued**

resources that could be rapidly mobilized in the event of another hurricane. This prior coordination caused the number of ambulance companies who contributed to the response effort to reach more than 150. Ambulances from 35 states—50% of ground ambulances supplied by AMR's subcontracted network providers—responded to Mississippi, Louisiana, and Texas. Through prior communication and planning, AMR allowed for a nearly seamless approach to providing assistance to people during this catastrophic event.

---

## Factors Impeding Preincident Coordination

EMS preplanners should consider several issues as a part of coordination during the preplanning process. Autonomy of actions will sometimes prevent individual agencies from willingly taking on the responsibility of coordinating prior to an event or incident. An agency's desire to be duly recognized for its contribution to a response might also dissuade it from engaging in coordination with other response agencies. There might be a fear among responders that coordination will result in a loss of a particular agency's valuable resources. EMS organizations may also want to evaluate how they will benefit from coordination before making the effort to respond in cooperation with outside agencies.

### Autonomy of Actions

One of the most frequent impediments to coordination in preplanning is individual organizations' desire for autonomy of actions. For example, someone who has served in EMS and emergency response for 20 to 30 years tends to have an idea of what is going on and they may go and do what needs to be done when they deem it necessary. Such independent actions may prevent tasks from being completed or cause them only to be partially accomplished. During the preplanning process, it is important to remind the organization of the overriding goals during an incident: ensuring life and safety and treating patients with the best care the agency is able to provide.

### Credit and Recognition

Agencies may also fear that coordination will cause either an individual responder or the group to lose its identity. Responders and agencies want to know that they will be recognized for their efforts. Even when they are responding with mutual aid or acting as a secondary responder, they like to be identified and acknowledged for what they have done. Consider the following example: If a large fire or incident with multiple-town and multiple-agency response occurred and a particular response agency involved was not explicitly acknowledged in the press covering the incident, that agency's staff might become upset and refuse to respond to future incidents. Responders and agencies fear they will be lost in a major multiple-agency event and that they will not be given credit. After an incident, agency leaders should take the time to write a brief letter to assisting organizations' directors, thanking them for their response and assistance.

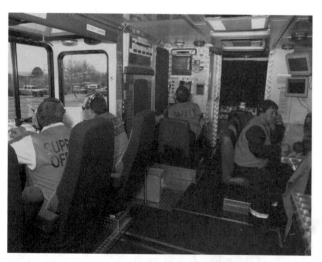

**Figure 9-1** Experience has shown that large-scale incident response failure is often the direct result of a lack of coordination between the involved emergency response agencies.

## Resource Allocation

Another issue of concern to agencies involved in multiple-agency responses is resource allocation or a loss of resources. Agencies sometimes feel that if they coordinate, resources that make their organization unique will be diverted for another, unintended use. The loss of that resource, they believe, will also lead to a loss of identity. To prevent this diversion of resources, prior communication among agencies will need to take place outlining the who, what, when, where, and how of resource allocation.

## "What's In It for Me?"

A corollary to the previous concern is a perceived lack of benefit. Organizations may feel that they have nothing to benefit from coordinating. By having strong mutual aid agreements in place prior to an incident, organizations will know that the lead agency will be there for them when they need assistance. Contributing agencies, in turn, will offer their services in the coordinating agency's time of need.

EMS agencies need to be cognizant of and deal with factors that impede coordination. Organizations may need to manage the concerns of their personnel multiple times before lasting change occurs. It is hoped that the agencies and individuals being called to coordinate through the preplanning process will realize the benefit of incorporating coordination into preplanning efforts. The goal of more efficient responses to major incidents should motivate increased cooperation and enthusiasm for the tasks associated with preincident coordination.

# Facilitating Coordination

The process of coordination is made easier when the involved agencies share their goals and expectations for preplanning. Having common leadership for the preplanning effort among multiple agencies can also facilitate interagency coordination. During the process of preincident coordination, it is also helpful for agencies to communicate their needs to one another, to enhance each organization's ability to support the others.

## Shared Goals and Expectations

Establishing a common set of preplanning goals and expectations will allow agencies to work together more efficiently. This has held true from kindergarten all the way through public policies and work laws; bringing people together works better than separating them. Defining a set of goals prior to an incident will allow for all individuals and organizations involved to know what is expected of them, and what they can expect in return.

## Shared Leaders

Having shared preplanning leaders between involved agencies can facilitate coordination. A regional advisory council, for instance, is made up of members and leaders from multiple response organizations and multiple disciplines. Regional advisory council members may have close ties to outside agencies; these ties will facilitate response coordination. Leaders of the regional advisory council may work in fire, EMS, or law enforcement. Within the council, however, there may also be potential contacts to hospital administration, which may be able to provide guidance or oversee the coordination effort.

## Shared Needs

The last major issue impeding coordination is similarity of resource needs. As was mentioned earlier, EMS organizations may be afraid of losing their resources, which they feel could also result in a loss of identity. When coordinating agencies see that the involved agencies have similar needs, they are more likely to help coordinate their available resources, while maintaining their identity.

# Benefits of Coordination

In order to move past the impediments to coordination, EMS agencies must realize that coordination is a beneficial activity for every organization involved. The benefits of coordination include legitimized response actions, increased response availability, continuity of care for patients at the incident scene, as well as organizational pride.

### Legitimacy of Action

Coordination, or the process of working with others towards a common goal, gives legitimacy to the response effort. One of the things that EMS has seen in action reports from around the world, through the World Health Organization (WHO), is that when legitimacy of actions breaks down—either from lack of planning or lack of communication—a mistrust develops between all agencies involved. By working together, all involved response agencies share the benefit of legitimized response action.

### Increased Response Availability

Decreased duplication of effort, due to interagency coordination, results in increased response availability and utilization. When EMS agencies cooperate, they are less likely to use the same resources or perform identical response actions. One of the issues from Hurricane Katrina, and from September 11th, was that multiple agencies should have enough ambulances; ambulances were provided, but were not always the vehicles that were needed. Sometimes buses were needed but ambulances showed up because there was a communication breakdown. Taking these past failures into consideration, when agencies coordinate, they should know what resources are needed and not to send ambulances when they are not needed. This will allow people that need ambulances to have access to them, while providing those needing buses with the appropriate transportation.

### Continuity of Care

Another benefit of coordination is continuity of care. When incidents occur, responders must mitigate patients' emotional and physical suffering to the greatest extent possible. The extent of this suffering is contingent upon the quality of care that the patients receive. A decrease in human suffering occurs when EMS agencies coordinate their actions. Through preplanning for continuity of care, patients are able to receive adequate medical attention in a timely fashion.

### Organizational Pride

When coordination results in an efficient response to a major incident, responders from the involved agencies can say of themselves, "We were part of that; we accomplished what was needed. We did a good job." Efficiency of response through interagency cooperation helps organizations to achieve pride. This is a positive influence, helping later on with recruitment, retention, and funding. Having proof that the agency is capable of doing its job well provides outside donors with funding rationale.

# Logistical Considerations

EMS agencies must coordinate the following logistical aspects of emergency response with all involved response organizations: staffing, use of the physical space available at an incident scene, use of equipment or other resources, and funding for the response effort.

## Staffing

A cooperative response effort requires coordination of each agency's staff. Planners must determine the appropriate staffing levels to respond to an incident. During transportation of patients and resources, for instance, which personnel will be involved? Will it be necessary to rotate the staff after so many hours? How will these personnel be provided for?

Since the impacts of Hurricanes Katrina and Rita, several nursing home corporations have begun to look at taking care of their staff and staff-member families. Then, when preplanning for evacuation, they not only look at taking residents and certain staff members out, but also incorporate staff-member families into the evacuation plan. Including the immediate families of staff members in the evacuation process adds a benefit to the staff involved of not having to worry about the safety or location of their families.

## Physical Space

Coordination of space must occur during preplanning for incidents requiring a response from multiple agencies. Planners need to determine where to set up operations and the incident command post (see **Figure 9-2**). Each EMS agency's role in the ICS must be coordinated prior to the response effort. The involved organizations must also understand their span of control in different areas at the incident scene: Do they play a significant role in incident command, and therefore have control over other EMS agencies' on-scene operations? Do they direct activity in the emergency room (ER)? What other patient care areas will require EMS supervision, and who will oversee them? Whoever is in "control" is responsible for staffing designated physical spaces at the scene of the incident. Agencies may also be delegated responsibility for ambulances, buses, or certain rooms within a building.

## Equipment and Resources

Equipment must be coordinated, as well. Consider the following example: There was an incident where a hospital had lost power, and they had lost backup generators. They had to call for EMS agencies to arrive to facilitate cardiac monitoring of patients because the power and backup were out. In cases such as this, equipment utilization must be coordinated.

It is important for agencies to determine how certain required equipment will be used during evacuation or while transitioning from the field to a receiving facility. When a patient attached to a monitor must move from facility "A" to facility "B," should the patient be detached from the monitor, connected to a transport monitor, or transported with the monitor from facility "A?" EMS agencies need to coordinate supplies utilized from facilities, or other agencies, and outline protocol for returning certain pieces of equipment to their original owners.

## Funding the Response

Before an incident or event, administration must coordinate who is going to pay for the information systems to be implemented, staff to provide care for patients, as well as physical spaces where the staff may work. The origin of funds for the equipment used in the physical space by the staff for the sharing of response information is usually handled in the early stages of preplanning.

In disasters considered "presidential-declared disasters" or emergency actions (as dictated in the Stafford Act), once a presidential declaration has been

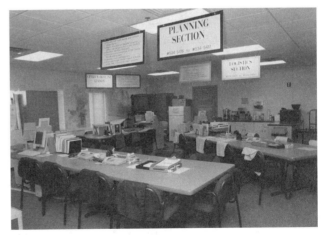

**Figure 9-2** An incident command system needs to be set up for large-scale terrorist and mass-casualty events.

### The Stafford Act

The Stafford Disaster Relief and Emergency Assistance Act (Stafford Act) is a US federal law designed to bring an organized and systemic process to federal natural disaster assistance for state and local governments in carrying out their responsibilities to aid citizens.

It created the system in place today by which a presidential disaster declaration of an emergency triggers financial and physical assistance through FEMA. The Stafford Act gives FEMA the responsibility for coordinating government-wide relief efforts.

made, it is the responsibility of the Federal Emergency Management Agency (FEMA) or the federal government to pay for most, if not all, response needs.

# Requesting Outside Assistance

Now that general considerations associated with preincident coordination have been addressed, this chapter will take a closer look at how determination of response needs is linked with working in cooperation with other local and federal agencies to achieve preplanning goals. The first area EMS agencies look at prior to coordination with other agencies and organizations is the capabilities of local facilities or the venues that they are planning for. Necessary details include who is present at the facility or venue, what potential hazards or possibly useful resources are stored there, when the event or incident will occur, where incident command can be set up, and how agencies may most efficiently respond. As described in chapter 3, responders collect this information through assessments and from the facilities themselves before developing a response plan. In conducting hazard, risk, and gap analyses, EMS agencies are able to look at coordinating times, trigger points, transition, and continuity of care. Once the appropriate details have been determined, EMS may move forward with response coordination with other agencies.

### Local Response Agencies

EMS should first look into coordinating with other response agencies. This may include the fire department if they are not part of EMS, local law enforcement, or other emergency response organizations. It is important for EMS agencies to ask: Who is nearby that may provide assistance? Such organizations are usually found within the city's municipality jurisdiction. After considering local agencies, preplanners can look to other important agencies such as public health, parks department, and possibly transportation. These other organizations, however, may not be traditional response agencies and may need considerable guidance to support EMS. This may be a challenge, but identifying what is needed and why it is needed will help the nontraditional response agency to support EMS.

### Local Resources

Local resources such as public health and transportation are usually requested through command channels, either directly by the incident commander or through an emergency operations center (EOC). By coordinating with these local resources, EMS gains a quicker and better-prepared response. For example, in certain cities, the public health department has decontamination capabilities and will respond to large hazardous materials incidents. The public health department also may provide EMS agencies with physicians, nurses, technicians, equipment, and methods for monitoring patients.

The transportation department can provide EMS agencies with vehicles such as buses. They may also make carry-all vans available to agencies in need of them.

The parks department can bring tents, chairs, and tables to an incident scene. They may also be able to provide space, such as public parks or venues, which may be accessed and used by emergency personnel during a response.

The streets department can assist emergency response agencies with barricading or channeling the flow of traffic or coordinating to have an avenue or route set up for ambulances and EMS personnel to access the incident site.

## Mutual Aid Agencies

Mutual aid is the most common contact that EMS agencies make to request assistance. Usually this assistance comes from nearby agencies such as fire departments and other EMS organizations. Though it is also common to look to other fire, EMS, or law enforcement agencies for assistance, when agencies plan for mutual aid, they need to coordinate a total response of assets within their organization, resources within their jurisdiction, as well as the external assets that are available to them. Mutual aid is usually requested from the incident commander through the dispatch center or other EOCs with a specific request of what is needed, where it is needed, and for approximately what length of time it is needed.

## Emergency Operations Centers

Another place to consider when beginning coordination is the EOC. An EOC will have a list of resources and points of contact for issues that may arise, both during preplanning and throughout the incident. They know what contractors are available and can assist in making arrangements for purchase orders or for quick turnaround of supplies. They know who has what resources (perhaps in a neighboring jurisdiction), and they will supply the appropriate contact information so that EMS agencies can coordinate with them for what they need, as identified through hazard, risk, and gap analyses. Hazard or risk analyses identify the potential hazards associated with an incident, event, or facility. A gap analysis objectively examines what is needed and what is on hand to deal with hazards facing an EMS agency.

EOCs will also know the community-wide response plan for a given incident, facility, or event. They more than likely drafted it or had a significant part in its development, and they will have information about what has been done in the past. EMS agency coordination with the EOC can prevent duplication of response effort. For instance, if the EOC has already coordinated through public health and the Department of Transportation (DOT) for their functions, it saves agencies the step of doing the same in preparation for a response. For this reason, it is beneficial for EMS agencies go through at least the initial contact with the EOC.

## Community Emergency Response Teams

One overlooked area of coordination is the community response with a community emergency response team (CERT), the citizens fire academy, and citizens police academy. These groups are made up of civilians who volunteer their time to assist the community. EMS agencies often do not consider what these organizations have to offer, because they are not directly involved with the patient care. These agencies, however, may be quite valuable for responding to a long-term incident. They may be able to assist EMS, for instance, with setting up rehabilitation sectors. They may offer additional personnel to oversee administrative tasks. These agencies may be able to offer ham radio operators or other telecommunicators that are willing to assist. These people are out there and are willing to help; CERTs are a great resource because they are volunteers who have already stepped up to the plate to offer assistance in times of need. EMS should consider coordinating the involvement of volunteers, in a way that ensures that they are not harmed during the emergency response.

## Civic Organizations

Similar to community response agencies, civic agencies or organizations also employ volunteers. A civic organization could be the local Elks Lodges, Masonic Lodges, Moose Lodges, or scouting organizations.

> **Emergency Operations Center**
>
> An EOC is a centralized, protected location from which the emergency manager or municipal executive directs emergency operations and provides support to on-scene incident management. EOC "liaisons" or representatives assigned to the EOC provide input and reports to the emergency manager and provide support tasks to their agencies. EOC liaisons are normally organized by their emergency support function such as law enforcement, fire suppression, public utilities, public health, etc.

Great projects for coordination can be accomplished with Eagle Scouts, for instance, because they volunteer their time and may be able to set up some response functions. Certain civic organizations may be able to offer assistance beyond an EMS agency's capabilities or at a lower price, due to the group's preestablished connections with outside emergency response agencies. For these reasons, civic organizations are a great resource and should not be disregarded during EMS preplanning.

## Local Government Administrators

It can be beneficial for EMS agencies to coordinate with the city or county they serve by communicating with jurisdictional management, the mayor, county commissioners, the city planner, or the city manager. Contacting other agencies within the city (eg, the EOC, city management) adds some credibility to the preplanning effort. Also, those within an EMS organization who are hesitant to contribute to preplanning can be persuaded of its worth if, for example, the city manager or the mayor gives his or her seal of approval: "It is really great that this is happening. We would love it if your personnel participated to the fullest extent possible." These stakeholders get buy-in and also help encourage buy-in from other agencies. This is discussed in more detail in chapter 11: Administration.

## Private Companies

Private companies local to an EMS agency's jurisdiction are also an excellent resource and should be coordinated with in preparation for large-scale incidents. Consider the following case study.

### Case Study

The response effort during Hurricane Katrina extended from many places in the country. In the author's home city of Garland, TX, there was a great need for assistance of most every kind to support evacuees. Local and national chain pharmacies and retail stores were very willing to assist in helping out as much as possible. Free medication prescriptions and refills were given to evacuees once they saw the local public health physician at one of the mobile public health clinics set up by the public health department and fire department. Additionally, civic organizations and churches provided places to sleep, housed families for several weeks, and provided meals for evacuees.

Certain stores may be able to provide camping gear, such as air mattresses or pads so that emergency care providers can make laying on backboards easier for patients. Bus companies may offer their services to help with transportation of people in an emergency; they can actually use their involvement as a tax write-off for donated time and equipment. Equipment rental agencies may have multiple generators, water pumps, or other equipment EMS agencies may need, depending on the facility or the venue being preplanned for. Finally, EMS agencies can look at home health agencies. These include a variety of health care providers, from nurses to technicians, who have had experience providing care to patients. They also often have resources to provide care to large amounts of patients, as well as various oxygen delivery devices such as oxygen generators. Enlisting their support can be very valuable. This is especially true when considering geriatric or special needs populations, where home health care providers will really be in their element. Home health agencies may volunteer their time or services or be a source of coordination. Typically, home health organizations are known to EMS organizations prior to an incident, and often assistance is just a phone call away.

## Outside Volunteers

It is also important for EMS agencies to look at potential volunteers such as members of medical societies, students, nursing professionals, people who work in pharmacies, or paramedics in training that may be able to volunteer in some capacity. Many times during disaster response, the walking wounded or walking worried patients outnumber those who are truly injured. Having medically trained people available can assist an EMS agency to prioritize patient care while addressing the concerns of all people affected by an incident. When these types of volunteers arrive at the scene of an incident, they should be directed to the designated liaison officer, to await further assignment.

## Coordinating With the Media

In the world today, it is important to coordinate effectively with the news media. This is, unfortunately, a double-edged sword. If an EMS agency coordinates effectively with the media, the media can increase interest and visibility in a project as well as the organization working on it. The benefit of having the news media cover a planning session, looking at the exact type of issue that just hit another community, will show that an agency is taking a proactive stance in preplanning. To those that an EMS organization serves, it shows that the organization is concerned and that it is making a concerted effort to provide effective care for the community (see **Figure 9-3**).

Increased publicity for an agency is an indirect benefit of coordinating with the media. Many times publicity leads to increased funding. It can also persuade hesitant personnel to shift from resistance to assistance in terms of preplanning. When the media shines a positive light on an organization's preplanning efforts, the emergency personnel and other emergency response agencies will see legitimacy in the tasks associated with preplanning. There is also a possibility that outside agencies' willingness to assist may be due to their desire to be seen as part of the agency's proactive efforts, because it will draw attention to the involved agencies. The more coordination an agency engages in, the more assistance it will be able to get. Coordination efforts should always be guided, however, by the higher goal of planning for the most efficient and effective emergency response.

## Methods of Coordination

After determining who an agency will coordinate with, it is next necessary to look at how this coordination will occur. Two types of coordination are possible: voluntary and directed.

### Voluntary Coordination

Voluntary coordination is obviously the better method of the two. It is more conducive to an organization, allowing for increased effectiveness in the coordination effort. A voluntary effort involves people who willingly offer their assistance and tend to seek out opportunities to donate their time and service.

### Directed Coordination

Directed coordination is almost equivalent to being drafted. Many times, recruited volunteers will only do

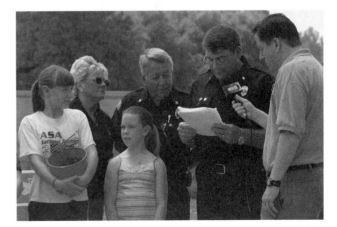

**Figure 9-3** Coordinating effectively with the media can aid in publicly demonstrating an EMS agency's involvement in the concerns of the community it serves.

enough to say that they have accomplished what was asked of them. The goal of an agency dependent upon the use of directed assistance is to convert the directed group into a voluntary one.

Directed help might include an agency that was resistant to the preplanning effort or the city manager that has now deemed your project a worthwhile cause. These resources will join the emergency response plan (ERP) development process, but will very likely be present only to do the minimum amount of planning. First, EMS agencies have to be cognizant of why people join this effort involuntarily: Is it because they feel forced? Is it in response to peer pressure or pressure from senior individuals? EMS agencies need to work with directed assistance as closely as possible. It is important for EMS to show that they are grateful for the support of these contributors: "We know that this is hard work and a considerable time commitment, but we really appreciate your assistance." If it is not possible to persuade directed help to become voluntary, the EMS organization may get the minimum effort that it needs.

# The Importance of Effective Communication

Communication, or the effective exchange of information, is critical when dealing with large or sensitive incidents. When preplanning for incidents, events, and facilities, it is imperative to predetermine what information will be needed by all agencies involved. In terms of response information, agencies must consider the source agency and other agencies who will be notified. EMS organizations must ask of themselves: How will information be communicated from one agency to another, one agency to multiple agencies, or to multiple facilities? Information sharing occurs between all agency levels: vertical and horizontal information feeds occur. Information goes up to command from individual functions of the incident, such as operations or planning, and direction comes down from command to the individual functions of the incident. The flow of information from the lowest echelon to the highest is important, so that decisions can be made at all levels with proper information.

An EMS agency can communicate in several ways for the purposes of preplanning, including via telephone or email, large informational meetings, and face-to-face meetings with coordinating agencies.

## Telephone and Email

Telephone and email correspondence can be useful for making initial contact with coordinating agencies and planning meetings. These modes of communication allow participants to juggle multiple tasks while remaining in contact with the necessary organizations. Although telephone and email are useful for communicating basic information, they do not allow EMS agencies to give the same personal attention to outside assistance as a face-to-face conversation. Emails are very easy to respond to, but may leave double meanings by the way the words or the sentences are crafted. Also, when people are on the telephone or reading emails, they can be distracted easily. Because such interactions are not face-to-face, the immediate call to action may be lost, and it could take longer to accomplish tasks necessary for effective preplanning.

## Informational Meetings

Although informational meetings are very efficient for disseminating large amounts of information to many people, they are slightly less personal than face-to-face meetings. These meetings provide an excellent opportunity for everyone involved to convene, but it is easier for people or organizational members to hide and not fully participate. As a result, EMS agencies may find that directed assistance will actually show up and take part in these meetings, but will still provide minimal preplanning support.

## Face-to-Face Meetings

Face-to-face meetings are the most effective. Their effects are long lasting, and they tend to hold more attention. People work face-to-face; businessmen have known for years that face-to-face meetings go a long way in establishing rapport and getting what they want. Given a choice between a teleconference or showing up for a business meeting for a million-dollar contract, most people will attest that a face-to-face meeting worked out best. These meetings allow both groups to see the faces, see the reactions, and understand each agency's needs on a human level. Face-to-face meetings, however, are also the most time-consuming because there is a lot of give-and-take and information sharing, both verbal and nonverbal. It is well worth it, however, if EMS agencies have the time to commit to making a personal connection with coordinating agencies prior to execution of a preplan.

This chapter has touched upon the process of determining who EMS agencies must talk to during preplanning coordination and explained the effectiveness of certain communication methods. Overall, it is important that all agencies involved in an emergency response communicate before the incident. Each organization must make an effort to be specific in sharing information and expressing its needs.

## Selected References

American Medical Response: *AMR Disaster Response Team Recent Disaster Responses: 2008 Hurricane Gustav and Hurricane Ike.* http://www.amr.net/getdoc/aa1290ab-3526-470c-8c39-07c6b9bc4d80/Recent-Disaster-Responses. aspx. Accessed December 1, 2009.

*FEMA 592: Robert T. Stafford Disaster Relief and Emergency Assistance Act, as Amended, and Related Authorities;* Washington, D.C., FEMA; June, 2007.

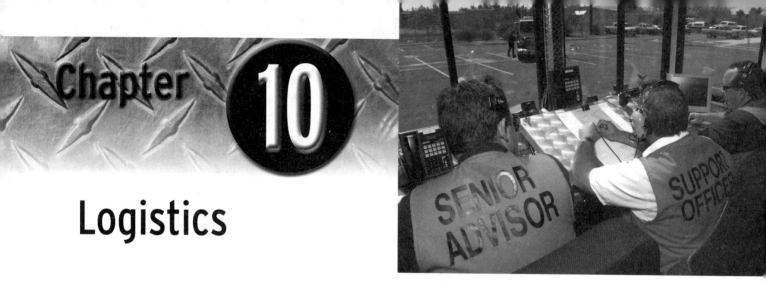

# Chapter 10

# Logistics

## Introduction to Logistics

What is the difference between a trauma surgeon in an ambulance and a paramedic in an ambulance (aside from obvious differences in education)? The answer is "none." Trauma surgeons without the equipment necessary to perform surgery, re-perfuse the patient, and address the myriad other equipment-related issues are care providers without the supplies to perform to their best ability. Similarly, EMS agencies without the equipment and supplies needed to perform their functions cannot properly take care of patients. Getting the right supplies to the ambulances to carry out their function is known as the process of logistics planning.

So, what is logistics? According to the National Incident Management System (NIMS), it is "providing resources and other services to support incident management." The military definition of logistics is "the science of planning and carrying out the movement and maintenance of forces... those aspects of military operations that deal with the design and development, acquisition, storage, movement, distribution, maintenance, evacuation, and disposition of material; movement, evacuation, and hospitalization of personnel; acquisition of construction, maintenance, operation, and disposition of facilities; and acquisition of furnishing of services." *Webster's Dictionary* offers yet another perspective, defining logistics as "... the procurement, maintenance, distribution, and replacement of personnel and material."

Formal EMS is still a relatively new phenomenon in relation to other medical operations. Although this text is about EMS, it is important to examine the long-term accounts of logistics. The historical perspective of logistics or "getting the right thing to the right place at the right

### Case Study

Unfortunately, almost every year the news is full of stories of wildfires in California. Units are mobilized and respond from all over the state to protect homes and towns from the flames. After the command function is established, one of the key support functions that is set up is the logistics function. This function establishes areas where equipment is staged, personnel are fed and can sleep, replacement parts can be retrieved, and other essential tasks of the overall operation occur.

As it is with wildland fires, so it is with large EMS operations. Hurricane Katrina is another recent example of large logistical support of a large operation. Warehouses and truckloads of medical supplies, fuel, water and other miscellaneous supplies were established to support the massive efforts of the response.

time" is replete with excellent examples during military operations.

Military victories, much like successful emergency medical services (EMS) incident responses, depend on logistics—this has been proven time and time again, throughout history. In World War II, German Field Marshal Erwin Rommel established a supply line that started in Italy and ran through Tunisia. He was defeated by Allied forces because his logistic line was cut. Also, during the 1944 D-Day landings at Normandy, the Allies planned for and maintained an adequate and robust logistics arm; this was one of the critical factors that led to their eventual victory. These events, although military and not EMS in nature, prove that logistics play a critical part in the successes and failures of large-scale operations (see **Figure 10-1**).

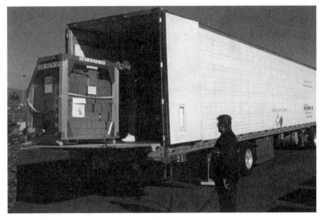

**Figure 10-1** Logistics planning can make or break a large-scale emergency response.

Modern disaster response, such as the response employed during the 2008 midwestern US floods, also exemplifies the need for adequate logistics. A lack of preplanning for resources and support allowed water to flow inside the affected regions. In response to the flooding that occurred throughout the Southwest in 2006, however, a strong, well-planned logistics initiative provided sandbags, wood, and other building materials responders needed to control the floodwaters.

## Assessing Current Logistics Capabilities

When planning an emergency response, the logistical questions are numerous; answering these questions is a major component of the preplanning process. It is essential for agencies to understand the logistics capabilities of their emergency response system as part of the preplanning process. The following must be determined: Does the agency have enough supplies, manpower, and equipment available to handle an incident or event? If not, where will it acquire these assets? Where will these assets be stored and prepositioned? Once these questions have been answered, an agency is equipped to establish protocol for storing and distributing supplies.

In general, there are two types of supplies: basic life support (BLS) and advanced life support (ALS). BLS supplies are needed for BLS skills and include bandages, adhesive bandages, suction equipment, and oxygen masks. ALS supplies support the utilization of ALS-level skills and can include IV supplies (such as IV catheters), medications, pharmaceuticals, and pads for defibrillators or monitors. Supplies can also be broken down into the categories of durable, expendable, and capital equipment.

Durable equipment is usually equipment that is made to be used more than one time, but it may have a wear-out point, where after so many uses it is no longer viable. Expendable typically describes any supply that is consumed for one patient contact, such as tape, an IV starter kit, or even an oxygen mask.

Capital equipment generally describes large-scale purchases, which cost a great deal of money. Agencies will invest in capital supplies one at a time. A cardiac monitor and a new ambulance are good examples of capital acquisitions. Most agencies will designate a fixed dollar amount within the budget to capital supply purchases, while others will allow a certain quantity of supplies. This equipment must to go through the capital budget in order to be replaced. Durable and expendable supplies, on the other hand, may be listed in the preplanning budget underneath a broad category, such as "medical supplies." Then, a purchase order will be used to secure all supplies listed under that heading.

## Supply Storage Systems

There are generally two different types of supply storage systems: centralized and decentralized. A centralized storage system describes a single facility where all materials for an agency are stored. A decentralized storage system is a series of multiple, smaller material-storage locations.

### Centralized System

The benefit of having a centralized location for the storage of an agency's supplies is that a central location is easier to control. It facilitates accounting for materials as they come in and out of the supply location. Few EMS agencies and fire departments utilize one central storage point, however, in part because fewer people at one time may have access to the supply facility. One major concern with regard to the utilization of a centralized supply location is that it lessens the overall flexibility of an agency to respond or to adapt when an emergency situation changes. Access to the material may be limited to just a few key people, and then access to the material becomes contingent upon the availability of those few personnel to unlock the storage facility and distribute supplies. Centralized supply storage may be feasible, however, for organizations with minimal personnel.

Traditionally, a very controlled delivery method—one that is dependent upon emergency providers' requests for additional supplies—is used to send supplies from a centralized logistics area to the point of impact, where resources are needed. This method has the potential to slow down or hinder overall operations as it is contingent on knowledge of what supplies are available as well as a preexisting communication system. Because centralized storage can hold larger quantities of supplies, EMS agencies should work stock rotation into daily operations in order to avoid expiration of medical supply packaging and gas-sterilized packaging. A centralized storage area may also be compromised due to the nature of an incident. For instance, the main facility might be surrounded by water or taken out by a tornado and be rendered inaccessible. It may then become an Achilles' heel for the operational aspects of the organization.

### Decentralized System

A decentralized supply system may consist of two or multiple logistics resupply points; these points may be located at agency substations or other geographically appropriate facilities strategically placed throughout the EMS agency's response area. Another example of a decentralized storage area is a disaster supply cache. Decentralized storage areas provide more flexibility for organizations by storing supplies closer, in most cases, to the people requiring those supplies.

A common concern with regard to decentralized systems is that the disparate locations of an agency's storage areas may result in decreased control over stock. Without a method of accountability, it is more difficult to keep track of inventory for a decentralized supply system. As a result, there is a better chance that pilferage and misuse of supplies will occur. **Table 10-1** lists the advantages and disadvantages of centralized versus decentralized supply systems.

## Supply Distribution Systems

In many instances, facilities that have a central logistics flow have fixed days or dates for resupply, such as on a certain day of the week or month. Disbursement may also occur at a station or substation of resupply points. This method is commonly used for the distribution of expendable supplies, which may be provided through an agreement between a hospital's emergency department and an EMS agency. An agency's dependence on such aid must be

**Table 10-1** Centralized Versus Decentralized Supply Systems

| Centralized Supply System | | Decentralized Supply System | |
|---|---|---|---|
| **Advantages** | **Disadvantages** | **Advantages** | **Disadvantages** |
| • Easier to control<br>• Facilitates resource tracking<br>• Suitable for EMS agencies with fewer personnel | • Fewer personnel may access at one time<br>• Decreased flexibility of response<br>• Very controlled supply delivery method<br>• Stock must be rotated regularly<br>• May be compromised during an incident | • Increased flexibility of response<br>• Resources stored in strategic locations, closer to response areas | • Resource tracking is more difficult<br>• Increased chance for pilferage and misuse of supplies |

carefully controlled, however, to avoid penalty under the "kickback laws" associated with use of Medicare monies. If an EMS agency brings patients to certain emergency departments, for instance, EMS may be able to restock without cost. These cost-free supplies may be seen as an inappropriate incentive (or "kickback") to bring patients to a particular hospital. Substations may also have limited stock availability and, as such, they may only store a limited number of a particular item.

A centralized supply location, on the other hand, will have greater quantities of the same item. Still, a substation may be adequate for a smaller location, such as an individual fire station. Other common examples of the decentralized supply model include ambulance stations or bases. These have small supply rooms or closets allowing supply storage for 1 or 2 weeks. Supplies may be kept on shelves as well as within the ambulance(s).

Station or substation resupply points are dependent upon a central supply for their resupply. In other words, responders must gather the appropriate resources from one central location. Supplies, in many instances, are sent to one central supply point, then are sent out to the multiple supply points.

### Readily Available Supplies

The types of supplies available to responders depend on the facilities in use. A large warehouse, for instance, will have a large storage capacity. A large warehouse accommodates a large inventory, but will usually require a large expenditure of funds as these supplies are bought in bulk. Traditionally, this has meant that certain items that are seldom used will be kept in storage for a period of time. As computer tracking of supplies comes into favor, however, EMS has the ability to track items more effectively. This allows those in charge of resupply to purchase specific items in a timely manner, eliminating the potential for purchasing an excess of unnecessary supplies.

Depending on the size of an EMS agency, there may be validity to the mass purchase and storage of certain supplies in a centralized location or large warehouse. A few smaller, neighboring EMS agencies may decide to purchase supplies as a group, so as to ensure standardization for mutual aid and to decrease the cost to each individual agency. Using a centralized storage location for resupply may entail some increased complexity in standard procedure, depending on the size of the additional facility. One of the benefits of this method, however, is that it usually affords the EMS agency a certain amount of redundancy. An agency would have multiples of an item in stock, and in the case of a large-scale incident, they would have the ability to push many or all of these items out to the end user.

### Just-in-Time Delivery

"Just-in-time" delivery is a method of supply delivery where items are ordered and delivered as needed, rather than stocked at the EMS agency. This manner of delivery has come into favor, because EMS agencies are more dependent upon computers to perform many daily or routine tasks, including tracking their supplies. The use of computers allows the agencies to maintain databases, to better track supplies and call up purchase orders for individual supplies as they are needed. This is the norm in most businesses today. With the reality of 1- to 2-day shipping, "just-in-time" delivery is beneficial for the ordering of specific items, and it decreases overhead costs because there is less on-hand stock necessary. An agency can prepare for a variety of potential incidents and events, without purchasing every piece of equipment needed for the responses developed during preplanning. As a result, there is no need for an agency to have, own, repair, and maintain a centralized facility. Fewer personnel will be needed to oversee storage and distribution of supplies; the absence of an additional facility makes these tasks easier to manage.

One issue with "just-in-time" delivery is that it usually does not have redundancy or surge capacity built into the system. When an agency preplans for certain large-scale events that have the potential to become mass-casualty incidents (MCIs), it is a good idea to have redundancy built into the established supply system. A decreased ability for redundancy will make an organization more dependent on vendors to supply and arrange for delivery of items to the EMS agency. Incorporating "just-in-time" delivery into an agency's preplan will take away some flexibility of response.

### Order on Demand

A third type of supply delivery system is called "order on demand." This delivery system is typically used by smaller EMS agencies that field fewer calls and use certain supplies and materials infrequently. Smaller EMS organizations tend to purchase and have delivered only what they use on a frequent basis, and they tend to do so right after responders have used the last of the agency's existing supply. These smaller agencies must take this into consideration when preplanning.

## Logistics Preplanning

Logistics are the key to any operation, whether handled by an EMS agency, fire department, law enforcement entity, or even the military. For this reason, the incident command system (ICS) devotes an entire branch to logistics. Current methods of resupply directly influence how an agency preplans for a broad spectrum of incidents. Consider the following example: An EMS agency must preplan for the inauguration of a local elected official. The agency serves a major city, and the turnout for the inauguration is expected to be very big. It is necessary to perform a strengths, weaknesses, opportunities, and threats (SWOT) analysis as a component of preplanning for the event.

### SWOT Analysis

A SWOT analysis identifies a given agency's strengths, weaknesses, opportunity, and threats. It also looks at internal and external factors influencing the agency's capabilities. Considering the importance of logistics in preplanning, it becomes critical to have the logistics section involved in the early stages of emergency response plan (ERP) development. Some questions that will need to be answered in a logistical SWOT analysis include:

- What is the strength of the current system of delivering various types of supplies to the end users, paramedics, or EMS agencies involved in this event's ERP?
- Will there be a time delay for delivery of supplies in the event of an incident?
- Is there an opportunity to improve the established supply system before an event or response?
- If something were to occur at this event, what might be demanded of logistics?
- If a flood or some other large, adverse event were to arise, would it shut down the agency's planned response?

In SWOT analysis, an EMS agency must take a long, hard look at its logistical capabilities. Logistics should be prepared to answer honestly about what it is doing well, what it is not doing well, and what needs to be changed about the established supply system. While performing a SWOT analysis, it is important to keep several things in mind concerning the supply system in use:

- How do crews get resupplied?
- Where do responders go for supplies and how do they get them?
- How do crews get resupplied in adverse weather or on the weekends? Is the same system used? Is no system available? Is delivery available? Will crews need to call someone else in the agency who will have access to the supply system?
- How do crews communicate the need for supplies?
- Is there a form that has to be filled out? Will a telephone call to logistics suffice?

Every organization employs formal and informal processes. A SWOT analysis allows an EMS organization to evaluate each procedure and identify proper and improper ways of providing logistical support. Simultaneously, while going through the SWOT analysis, a gap analysis program will indicate where opportunities and threats exist within an agency's existing logistics branch.

---

### GAP Analysis

A good method to determine what may be needed is the use of gap analysis program (GAP). A gap analysis is an objective examination of what is needed and what is on hand to deal with a specific issue or a combination of issues facing an EMS agency. The gap analysis will indicate where opportunities and threats exist within an agency's existing logistics branch. Gap analyses need not be very complicated endeavors but should be as thorough as possible to address all potential issues. These include:

- *Need.* For each need, what is available and what is not?
- *Potential.* What is the potential for a given incident or event to occur?
- *Impact.* What will happen if the need is not met?

These questions define the gaps. An example of GAP analysis is when an EMS agency asks what the potential need is for a particular supply, such as IV tubing, in a disaster, and how many the agency has. EMS should identify a need, understand what may occur if that need is not met, and then proceed to develop a mechanism or process to meet the need.

To follow up on the findings from each of these analyses, it is necessary to determine when an agency will have the opportunity to improve its system. The practice of regularly evaluating existing logistical procedures and modifying them as needed paves the way for a more efficient preplanning process.

## Planning for Problems

After conducting SWOT and GAP analyses, an agency must plan for logistics-related problems. This step consists of analyzing potential preplanning roadblocks relating to incident complications and surge that may place stress on a logistics initiative. Such a roadblock occurred in the spring of 2009 with the H1N1 influenza when some EMS agencies failed to plan in their vendor agreement for a surge of masks and other expendable medical supplies as the nationwide demand suddenly spiked.

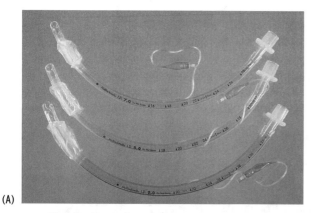

(A)

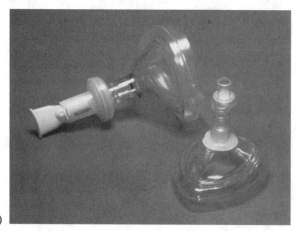

(B)

To begin, an agency must ask itself if it has a basic knowledge of how many supplies are used in its existing supply system on an average day, week, or month. Furthermore, an EMS organization should know how many of those available supplies are ALS, how many are BLS, and how many are expendable supplies (see **Figure 10-2**). To be thorough, an agency might analyze specifically how much tape, how many IVs, and how many oxygen masks are used on a regular basis. A base knowledge, or estimated inventory, of what is in stock and at what rate each item is consumed will provide a foundation for efficient logistical preplanning.

This base knowledge is also useful when some of the tougher questions concerning logistics' role in preplanning present themselves, such as:

- How will a 10% increase in calls or patients change logistical needs or the planned operational procedure?
- What if that 10% increase took effect over the course of 1 day? Over 1 week?
- Will a 20% increase in calls or patients change resupply methods? If so, how?

Once again the key to accurately answering these questions is to first address what SWOT and GAP analyses conclude about the vulnerabilities of the established supply and resupply system, so that the emergency response plan (ERP) can be modified. The next step is to determine what needs to be accomplished in terms of preplanning, to ensure the answer for the modified ERP will be, for example, "No, a 10% increase in calls or patients will not affect operations." A SWOT analysis helps identify issues that could arise during an incident or event that will derail the planned response or cause a surge. The 10%, 20%, or even 30% increase could represent additional patients from a car crash, plane crash, or from an overturned fertilizing truck containing gallons of

(C)

**Figure 10-2** It is important for EMS agencies to know what quantities of **(A)** ALS, **(B)** BLS, and **(C)** expendable supplies are available internally.

phosphate poisons, consequently increasing EMS patient load. If a surge or change in operations adds costs on top of its typical budget, an EMS organization will need to add the increase to its base number of runs and expenditures per day, to predict how the system will work in terms of budget.

## Preparing to Execute the Logistics Preplan

After an agency has assessed its plan for strengths and weaknesses, it is necessary to determine how the plan can be put into action. A system for notification needs to be in place, as well as a primary and a secondary method of getting supplies from the supply point to the crews. More importantly, a plan needs to be established outlining how the supply point will be resupplied as it distributes its stock.

When looking at two methods of resupply, the primary and secondary, it is important for an EMS agency to plan for effective notification of vendors as well as of those in charge of operations and logistics. If the central storage point has a depleted inventory, EMS personnel assigned to logistics will need to order more supplies. The request for resupply must be verified by the logistics section, and the vendor must also be able to support the need. If the vendor cannot provide an adequate supply, an agency may need to go to other vendors or a mutual aid municipality. The system cannot reliably count on help unless the message has been received and verified. It is dangerous to assume that a message has been received and understood. It is also dangerous to assume that the receiver will comply with the request. It is important to establish a protocol for making urgent calls, such as a request for resupply, to eliminate the possibility for error.

Dealing with vendors tends to complicate the process of requesting timely resupply. Remember, vendors have multiple customers. Some of these customers may also be EMS agencies, perhaps serving in the same region; they may even be a next-door neighbor. One vendor may have multiple customers requiring multiple services, all at the same time. This issue was really brought to the forefront of operations during Hurricane Rita when, for many EMS agencies in Texas, the resupply point were vendors that came out of Houston where they had large stocks of supplies stored in warehouses. Unfortunately, Houston was also hit by Hurricane Rita. The people responsible for moving supplies out to the agencies were not at work because they were evacuating. If there were a secondary vendor available to these agencies, the response to the devastation of Hurricane Rita would have been more efficient. A secondary vendor can be of great help in the event that a primary vendor experiences issues that preclude them from resupplying an agency's operation in a timely manner.

It is important to look at durable items that can be reused, as well as capital items, when preparing to contact a vendor. An agency can make an arrangement with the vendor for loaners, surge parts, or a small replacement part for a larger piece of equipment. It is important to take into account these small parts such as batteries for monitors, defibrillators, and cables. Cables often break or get lost on monitors. Having spare parts available with the vendor, who can push those to responders as needed, can be critical. When an agency buys equipment, it is actually possible for them to include the provision of these spare parts in the vendor contract. The agreement could say, for instance, in case of emergency the agency will be able to request a surge of "X" amount of parts. It is possible to identify the key spare components needed with the help of the manufacturer or the vendor.

---

### Preplanning Practices

An EMS agency may consider using a different region of the country for resupply access, as its secondary vendor. For example, if an organization's supplier is located on the East Coast, logistics for that agency may want its backup supplier to be based on the West coast. This would be a safe plan because the probability of the entire United States suffering a catastrophic failure of supply, communications, or transportation is minimal.

## Transporting Supplies

An EMS agency will also need to look at how they plan to manage moving supplies from one location to another. The agency's first consideration should be to assess the capabilities of the available storage location(s) and to plan for alternative supply storage sites. Having an alternative site for supply storage would enable responders to gather necessary supplies in the case of a flood, or other event resulting in blocked access. Having primary and secondary routes for delivery and distribution is critical. Once again, EMS must think operationally: When an agency considers evacuation, it must also incorporate evacuation into the response plan. Keeping the possibility of an evacuation in mind, an agency will decide that it needs to have a primary and secondary route in and out of the incident scene. One of the more important aspects of supply management is an EMS agency's ability to preplan for getting supplies to responders at the scene of an incident, as they are needed. If a delay presents itself (eg, flooding, adverse weather event, etc), having a plan in place allows resupply to occur. In the event that routes logistics normally takes to transport supplies are cut off, preplanning for an alternate route allows EMS and vendors to avoid blocked-off routes. The need for this form of preplanning was made apparent during Hurricane Katrina, when major routes of travel were affected. Bridges were out and traffic was clogged, making it very difficult for trucks to get in with necessary supplies.

Coordination of supply distribution in the face of operational road blocks is possible with the establishment of a primary and secondary plan. Transport of resources will be more difficult when bridges, tunnels, or other access routes are cut off, or when law enforcement sets up cordons to move people in and out of an incident scene. In response to that last example, an agency can coordinate with law enforcement, by alerting officials that EMS will have trucks for supplies needed to adequately respond to the emergency. If law enforcement knows these trucks will be coming through the main street, they can ensure supplies are able to get through. As seen here, communication with other agencies involved in the emergency response will only bolster an EMS organization's preparedness, in terms of logistics and resupply. Communicating with the vendor or the shipper is also important, to let them know what the best access routes will be for a given situation. These must be identified beforehand because, with preplanning, the more dependent an agency is upon "just-in-time" supply or service delivery, the more peoples' lives will be at risk for a given incident.

Utilization of loan agreements for various pieces of equipment with other emergency entities or vendors is also an important consideration during logistical preplanning. These loan agreements are similar to a form of logistical mutual aid. An EMS agency might be interested in forming a contract with another organization, to allow for use of its surplus supplies and equipment. Nearby agencies can coordinate together, to compile an overall inventory list. Then, as each agency determines its training, operations, and preplanning needs, interagency mutual aid can be coordinated. It is beneficial to find out what kinds of inventory nearby agencies have, in terms of equipment. Each agency should determine to what extent they may be able to assist another EMS organization and work that in as part of the loan agreements.

Lastly, it is important to coordinate with law enforcement to ensure that, as responders get additional supplies to the supply locations, the resources will be safe. This can be especially critical in cases of a bioterrorism attack when antidotes are coming in. In this case, logistics must ensure that the antidotes are delivered, processed by the system, given to the proper people, and are not pilfered from the loading docks, or from the truck.

## Logistics Preplanning for Long-Term Events

Logistical concerns for long-term incidents (incidents lasting longer than 72 hours) require a different preplanning approach. Incidents may carry on for days, such as Hurricane Katrina or the 2008 midwestern US floods. Incident command must be established and the various divisions and branches of ICS put in operation. One of the key areas in ICS during long-term incidents is logistics. Logistics is responsible for managing rehabilitation and rehabilitation locations; supply and eventual resupply of food and water; transport from staging areas to the incident location; shift changes; as well as movement of people back and forth to rest and rehabilitation areas. Long-term incidents require EMS organizations to preplan for sustaining a logistical supply over an extended period of time.

While emptying a warehouse and bringing everything in stock to the scene may work for small-scale incidents, this method is not a viable option for incidents lasting from one week to a few months. An EMS agency must consider how it will realistically deal with a long-term incident, given its inventory. The Federal Emergency Management Agency (FEMA) and other entities such as the Joint Commission on the Accreditation of Healthcare Organizations (JCAHO) have made it clear that any disaster will be handled by the local agency for up to 72 hours without outside assistance. This window of time is critical to bear in mind while preplanning for any incident. Emergency response agencies that are unable to self-sustain, whether through mutual aid or through its own mechanisms, will be out of operation when response efforts are needed most. Without adequate preplanning for various logistical and operational realities based on the aforementioned 72-hour window, the operation will inevitably become ineffective and shut down.

As a part of long-term planning, agencies should establish contingency contracts with multiple vendors to meet anticipated needs. During the responses to Hurricanes Rita and Katrina, even though many emergency response entities had preexisting contracts with supply vendors, when the hurricanes hit, vendors were stretched trying to supply so many agencies with the necessary supplies. Having the contingency of a secondary vendor in place is beneficial. An EMS agency may plan to request a push-pack containing specific items from vendor "A," for instance, but vendor "A" might be unable to make a timely delivery. A secondary plan might involve contacting vendor "B" who sells the same items, which will arrive on the scene only 24 or 48 hours behind schedule.

It is not realistic to expect a logistics preplan to account for all potential hazards and vulnerabilities at the scene of an incident. This is particularly true of responses to MCIs and sustained events; these types of incidents and events have the potential to quickly overwhelm what would be an adequate supply system for day-to-day operations. As the amount of casualties increases, however, an EMS agency has the opportunity to think ahead about what may be needed the most—a lack of supply preplanning should not become an Achilles' heel to an EMS organization.

An EMS preplan must address the importance of logistics, to ensure materials and supplies will arrive where and when they are needed. Because operational realities, staffing patterns, and other things change within an agency, logistical preplanning must be an ongoing process. It is safe to say that when logistical support fails, the EMS system fails. This is a truism that any army knows and can attest to. The US Army has 15 support personnel for every one infantryman in battle. This "long-tooth detail" affords the Army the ability to have sufficient supplies, equipment, and material moving forward and being replenished as it utilized. Some would argue that this ratio of support personnel to infantrymen has contributed to the US military's successes. EMS providers, managers, and systems need to engage in a similar philosophy in preplanning for a contingency, operation, or specific type of facility.

## Selected References

Arnold, J: Risk and risk assessment in health emergency management. *Prehosp Disaster Med* 2005;20(3):143–154.

Buerhaus, P and Staiger, D: Trouble in the nurse labor market? Recent trends and future outlook. *Health Aff*, 1999;18(1):1, 214–222.

Merriam-Webster Collegiate Dictionary. Springfield, MA: Merriam-Webster; 1961.

State of Missouri, State Emergency Management Agency: NIMS definitions and acronyms. http://sema.dps.mo.gov/ Planning/NIMS%20Definitions.doc. Accessed December 1, 2009.

United States Department of Defense: *Dictionary of Military and Associated Terms*. Joint Publication 1-02. April 12, 2001 (as amended through March 17, 2009).

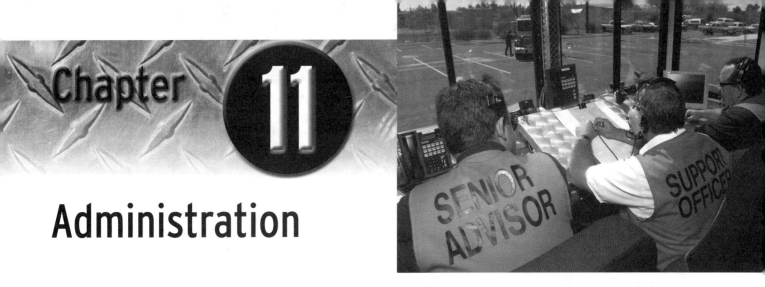

# Chapter 11

# Administration

## Administrative Buy-In and Support

To have a comprehensive emergency response plan, there must be administrative support. Just as a carpenter must construct a foundation before building a house, preparations must also be made to establish a working preplan. In building the foundation of a house, there are tasks that must be accomplished, such as framing the foundation and pouring the concrete. Similarly, an emergency response plan must be put into motion before an incident occurs. Consider the following scenario:

### Case Study

An emergency medical services (EMS) agency has an Amtrak train traveling through its response area. During preplanning, the organization asks the following questions: What will happen if the train derails, with 310 passengers on board? What plan will be in place, guiding responders to deal with victims? Will the agency need to request mutual aid? Will all responding units be allowed to freelance at the scene of the incident?

A comprehensive preplan must be developed to outline the steps that need to be taken when dealing with incidents. In preplanning, preparatory measures are essential. It is not enough to simply develop the plan in writing. Having the various preplanning elements in place will ensure an efficient emergency response when an incident occurs. By having the buy-in from administration, an agency will have the framework in place to assist in mitigating the incident.

## Proactive Leadership

Proactive organizational leadership is at the core of successful hazard mitigation. A proactive leader will take practical actions, to ensure the success of his or her team (see **Figure 11-1**). Some examples of practical actions include implementing the incident command system (ICS) at all incidents, regardless of size, and ensuring that all members of the organization have access to, understand, and incorporate the hazard plans. Many organizations commit to preplanning as a mechanism for improvement. Preplanning can become a catalyst for change within an organization, allowing for better-trained responders, increased situational awareness, and effective management of complex incidents.

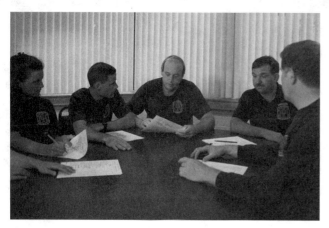

**Figure 11-1** Proactive leadership is essential for the success of any team.

A suitable sponsor within an organization may also provide proactive leadership to ensure preplanning is accomplished with minimal conflicts. The sponsor will essentially serve as the preplanning leader. This role may be taken on by the senior EMS officer. The officer must oversee the preplanning process to ensure that preplanning is accomplished and that major impediments are avoided or minimized.

Another key aspect of proactive leadership is having an informed and committed outside sponsor, such as senior local government officials (eg, hospital commissioner, mayor, etc), supporting the preplanning process. The outside sponsor needs to be informed of the need for preplanning (not only what resources are needed), but they must also understand the entire process and the potential catastrophic results that may occur if preplanning has not taken place. They must be strongly committed to accomplishing preplanning and participating in all of the activities that assist in the planning process to sustain the initiative. The outside sponsor will provide a clear mandate for the person who has been selected to move the process forward. In order to have effective preplanning, there needs to be strong and committed organizational leadership. Without committed leadership and outside sponsorship, the preplanning process will lack direction.

## Bringing Plans Together

The emergency preplan must tie in with the municipal strategic plan and supplement the county, regional, state, and national plans. An EMS agency must communicate with other key stakeholders, such as law enforcement and local fire departments, to ensure that there is one cohesive plan. A mutually consistent set of preplans allows each agency's resources to meld into a common operational team. If the plans are not mutually supportive or do not supplement the higher level plans, then external support will not be available for the planning process, nor will there be physical support for the enactment of the emergency response plan. Continuity of effort is essential.

A preplan must also be feasible and call upon available resources. An EMS preplan cannot plan for the local fire department to establish a decontamination area, for instance, if the fire department's preplan designates fire personnel the task of mitigating other potential hazards. Interagency cooperation is essential in scenarios such as this one, when responders are presented with patients requiring decontamination. Without effective communication between agencies, this vital step in patient care will be overlooked. This is counterproductive to the emergency response.

## The Preplanning Team
### The EMS Officer

One person must be charged with the task of ensuring effective preplanning. Preplanning should be the primary or the secondary job function of the EMS officer selected. EMS organizations should identify a key player within their department, and that person should be trained in the role of overseeing the preplanning process. In this way, the organization will maximize the productivity of the preplanning process by having someone in charge of mitigating work conflicts that interfere with effective preplanning.

## The Advisory Committee

An advisory committee or board can also be helpful for overseeing what is going on, acting as support for the agency's internal sponsor. The committee should meet at predesignated times or as needed. It may serve as a sounding board to bounce ideas and issues off of, while guiding the designated preplanning leader throughout the planning process. These committees are typically small groups of EMS individuals with an interest or background in the preplanning process and who have volunteered to be a part of the preplanning process. Committee members share their knowledge and experience with the designated preplanner, paving the way for the creation of a more accurate and concise preplan. The advisory board also provides a system of checks and balances, aside from providing procedural oversight.

## Administration Advocates

Besides having a designated EMS officer in charge of the preplanning process, it is beneficial to have an administration-level EMS advocate for the process. The function of this individual is to give credibility to the preplanning process, by including top-level management and agency leadership in the development phase. As with the advisory committee, administration-level advocates may share their expertise with the preplanning leader, to ensure efficient work is done. An administrative advocate serves as the EMS contact to a network of available resources; the advocate will know whom to contact for various situations that may arise during the preplanning process. This sponsor's expertise may be useful for maintaining contact with a National Transportation Safety Board (NTSB) representative in case of an airplane crash or a local structural engineer in the event of a building collapse. Whatever the need to accomplish the plan, the planner needs access to find answers, from prior fire preplans or access to the municipal plans or even the regional plans. This is actually where having an administration advocate is necessary. EMS agencies need someone with enough clout to get the planner the access needed and to express that need to other agencies' administrations.

# Identifying Preplanning Goals

It is important to identify preplanning goals. An EMS crew must first assess potential hazards and then determine how to mitigate them. It is necessary to examine both the strategic and tactical considerations. Responders should return to their hazard vulnerability analysis (HVA) to evaluate where the agency is heading and what needs to happen for it to get there. One technique that can be utilized in this phase of the preplanning process is the acronym GOSPA, which stands for the goals, objectives, strategies, plans, and activities.

GOSPA asks responders to first set an initial goal: "What is it that I want to accomplish?" Goal setting involves looking at short-, medium-, and long-term goals. Goals should include what needs be accomplished, why it needs to get done, what the team looks to accomplish by doing it, when it should be incorporated or implemented, and what it should look like once it is finished. Goals are the specific, long-term, measurable tasks that the team works toward accomplishing. Objectives are the short-term, internal goals that need to be met before the overall goal can be achieved. Strategy is a broad look at how one may best accomplish goals and objectives; plans outline step-by-step order of operations that individuals must take in order to achieve the desired objectives. Activities go hand-in-hand with

> **Preplanning Practices**
>
> EMS agency administration may use the acronym GOSPA to give direction to a preplanning effort:
>
> Goals
> Objectives
> Strategies
> Plans
> Activities

plans, detailing each person's responsibilities towards the achievement of a goal. This process begins with the end result in mind and works backward. In other words, knowledge of the overall goal will inform the deliberate process of evaluating what needs to be done in terms of objectives, strategy, plans, and activities.

# Evaluating Short- and Long-Term Planning

There is also a need to evaluate short- and long-term planning. EMS should evaluate how a plan will work in the short-term sense and assess how the plan will work in the future. Part of this involves doing a needs analysis. This is tied in with the HVA and core competencies of the agency. EMS will want to ensure that partnerships include all key stakeholders. These include those who have authority, are contributing resources, and are offering their expertise to the preplanning effort.

## Organizational Issues

Part of preplanning must involve the entire organization and the support of top-level management. Organizationally speaking, frontline people will never become enthusiastic or dedicated to the preplanning effort until they are treated as thinking people who are recognized as doing a good job and whose work is deemed important in achieving the overall goal. If frontline personnel present an idea for preplanning that is unrealistic or that the agency is unable to incorporate, for instance, management should inform personnel of why the suggestion is not feasible. Key operating processes will never work well unless department leaders also cooperate well with each other. This is true vertically and horizontally, between entities within the same organization as well as between organizations. Group buy-in must occur at all levels.

At a fire department-based EMS agency, for instance, preplanning is just as important, but may seem less exciting than firefighting operations. The organization must be proactive with preplanning, allowing all individuals to become actively involved in the process. Agencies must show that the vital work being done by the preplanning person is valued just as much as other operational issues. Typically, fire department operations are directed at saving lives and protecting property. If group buy-in has not occurred, then firefighters will focus on their main goals, but will not see the overall picture: that preplanning provides a basis for interdepartment cooperation and hazard mitigation.

# Plan Developmental Support

Once the individuals have been identified that will be participating in the preplanning process, the work of preplanning can begin. In order to plan, the required training and certifications must be obtained. Budgets must be allowed for these items.

## Learning to Preplan

After ensuring that the core group of individuals involved has been identified, the next key area that EMS needs to evaluate is the training and education for preplanning personnel. When discussing training and education for preplanning, there is a dearth of formal training that one can draw on. Preplanning per se is not taught in many institutions; typically, it is covered during on-the-job training. Agencies need to educate their personnel prior to starting the preplanning process as much as is practical. If there is a need to have a short turnaround, an education will not be possible; it must also be understood that most departments are not going to send someone to get a bachelors' degree in preplanning.

How does the agency provide specific education on preplanning? In many cases, they must contact experts in the field. These experts include local emergency management personnel, university personnel, and nationally known subject matter experts. Agencies may also obtain training from Federal Emergency Management Agency (FEMA) courses, such as IS-235 Emergency Planning, as a means to increase the planner knowledge base, or even lessons learned from various professional and government departments/agencies. Researching what is being planned for is also an effective preplanning tool. Responders may look into a particular event or facility, to find out whether a certain mission has been done before and to see how other people were able to mitigate the same or a similar emergency incident.

Professional resources such as the American Medical Association (AMA), Centers for Disease Control (CDC), FEMA, the International Association of Fire Chiefs (IAFC), International Association of Fire Fighters (IAFF), and International Association of EMS Chiefs (IAEMSC), each have position papers developed, best-practice guidelines, and numerous individuals with preplanning experience available for reference and guidance. All of these entities have valuable resources in planning for different issues, and many have other training/educational opportunities such as conferences and seminars.

In addition to the resources mentioned above, there are other organizations that have expertise from related perspectives. Hospitals, nursing homes, and the American Red Cross have disaster planning resources that may be beneficial for informing a preplanning effort. Although such information may not be directly related or may seem irrelevant, it is possible to take the principles from an outside agency's disaster planning resources and apply them to EMS preplanning. Nursing homes typically have disaster plans prepared for fires, pandemics, structural damage, or electrical failure. By reviewing their plan, the preplanner will be able to "see" the process from many different perspectives, incorporate relevant steps, and recognize potentially overlooked areas in the preplan being developed. One can also look at researching health delivery of some sort, public health hospitals, etc, as a guide to assist in various aspects of preplanning.

## Administrative Costs

Because costs will be attached and associated with preplanning, it is necessary for the administrative advocate to oversee the fiscal aspect of the preplanning process. It is not a good business or management model to have an operations chief directing someone to do preplanning if it is not budgeted through the operations section. When the preplanner or preplanning group is budgeted through another section, such as administration, without the person in charge of that section being aware of what is occurring, this creates conflict and may lead to misallocation of resources or even a failure of the preplanning process.

Ensuring the involvement of key stakeholders in the preplanning process can help to prevent budgetary issues. If the local police department is identified as a stakeholder, for instance, determining which department's budget will cover the cost of extra security and staffing can help to minimize fiscal discrepancies and promote unity.

## Certifications

One of the other kinds of issues involved with administrative costs may be additional or required certifications. Depending on what is being planned for, such as hazardous materials, it is mandated that the agency meet all applicable regulatory standards such as National Fire Protection Association (NFPA) Standards 471, 472, and 473. These certifications may add additional costs to cover training, physical examinations, and record maintenance. Additional insurance policies may also be required with the additional certifications.

If an EMS organization receives federal grant monies, the Department of Homeland Security (DHS) requires that the department become compliant with the National Incident Management

System (NIMS) (see **Figure 11-2**). While becoming NIMS compliant is an all-encompassing term, several specific aspects of compliance must be given attention: One aspect of NIMS compliance that DHS requires is for all responders be certified in IS-100 (Introduction to the Incident Management System), IS-200 (ICS for Single Resources and Initial Action Incidents), and IS-700 (NIMS An Introduction). While these courses are available free of charge from FEMA, additional department cost may be incurred as a result of this increased training requirement.

Another aspect of NIMS compliance is incorporating the Homeland Security Exercise and Evaluation Program (HSEEP) into an agency's yearly functional exercises. The HSEEP is a capabilities and performance-based exercise program that provides a standardized methodology and terminology for exercise design, development, conduct, evaluation, and improvement planning. The planner must be familiar with the HSEEP process, however, and may require additional certifications or training in order to properly execute a compliant exercise.

## Insurance Costs

Insurance costs will vary depending on the agency/organization, as well as the jurisdiction that is mandated to provide liability coverage. For some agencies, this may not be a significant issue, especially if the agency is a municipal entity. Most municipalities write a letter of self-insurance, stating that the municipality is acting as its own agent and has funds available for certain covered activities. If the organization is not a municipality, it may not be able to write such a letter of self-insurance and will therefore be dependent on gaining increased liability insurance commercially.

## External Costs

EMS personnel may choose to invest in computer software to assist with preplanning and associated issues. Certain programs are available that have been designed for fire preplanning and include photos and mapping, identification of known hazards, and incorporation of the preplan, and these programs may assist with EMS preplanning as well.

Another cost could be a consultant; it may be cheaper or more efficient to invest in this external expertise than to maintain internal expertise through software systems. The use of consultants may be a viable option, allowing for department-specific customization and incorporation, depending on the organization, how much preplanning they intend to do, and to what depth or level they are planning to do it.

## Benchmarks: How Is EMS Really Doing?

Benchmarking is crucial to the overall preplanning project. If the preplanning effort lacks direction, it will be impossible to validate the work done at any given point in the process. A team may find itself wandering aimlessly through emergency response plan (ERP) development and, worse yet, failing because of loss of resources resulting from inadequate scheduling.

Benchmarks are measurement tools that will allow a team to objectively compare costs, duration, productivity, or quality of a chosen action to one that is considered an industry standard. Benchmarks may detail specific items to be completed, time spent achieving the desired goals, or a combination of both. They can be determined based on directives for tasks relating to specific emergency response,

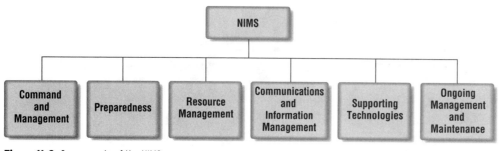

**Figure 11-2** Components of the NIMS.

through research of the events or incidents being planned for, or drawn from past experience with similar scenarios. Benchmarks employ a hierarchy of measurements to flesh out and provide a timeline for a team's action plan: high-, mid-, and low-level measurements. These are called detail measurements.

High-level measurements should relate directly to the organization's overall mission and goals. Hierarchy measurements need to be linked so that low- and mid-level measurements relate to higher-level ones. During the preplanning process, changes that occur in lower-level detail measurements—such as completing or being unable to complete an objective—will affect higher-level details in the work plan. In this way, the benchmark method of organizing and tracking preplanning efforts is very much akin to the GOSPA method mentioned earlier in this chapter. Either method would serve to maintain productivity in preplanning. Using the GOSPA method, if goals and objectives on the lower rungs are met, they should provide for efficient accomplishment of mid- and high-level goals and objectives.

Detail measurements should also relate to the most current and relevant systems and processes associated with emergency response. Having a plan that does not take into account the current system of operational guidelines and issues will not produce the most effective emergency response plan. The advisory committee must review the overall schedule as well as specific benchmarks, to ensure that things are being done in accordance with local policies and procedures before the work plan for preplanning is put into effect. Furthermore, each task associated with each detail measurement requires one person to be delegated responsibility for its completion—a point of accountability. This may be a single person or a group of people, such as a section.

Once benchmarks have been determined, they need to be validated by a team leader before they are used to guide those involved with the preplanning effort. Validation involves ensuring that the low-, mid-, and high-level details interact systematically to work toward the overall goal of preplanning. A team's schedule of benchmarks needs to reemphasize how the preplanning process will be organized. It is a good idea to have preplanning detail measurements plotted or displayed graphically and posted publicly, so that those involved in the effort can see where there is progress or a lack of progress. This allows everyone to understand where team focus needs to be, and how far along certain tasks are in relation to others. Sometimes called a dashboard, this tool allows team leaders to measure, publish, and evaluate preplanning progress.

# Personnel

When preplanning for an event, incident, or facility, an EMS organization must take into consideration the human resources available internally and the needs of those personnel. The number of responders available to carry out a response plan will determine the distribution of tasks, and it will also shape how ICS will be organized on the field. Additionally, assessing the current capabilities of an organization in comparison with the operations outlined in a given response will dictate what training and equipment the agency will need to invest in.

## Delegation of Authority and Span of Control

The planning leader may be tasked to report on the preplanning process to a different agency or to a different function within the agency. If the leader is tasked while functioning as the preplanning organizer, then the leader would be accountable to the outside group. It must be determined whether the leader will be accountable to the outside group on a full- or part-time basis. If he or she accepts full-time accountability to the outside group, responsibility for reporting must be fixed upon a single person or functional group, which should be held accountable for the success of the process. It is important to remember that the authority to perform a certain function can be delegated, while accountability cannot. As an example, if a chief who is accountable delegates authority for performing certain functions down to the captains and other people responsible, the chief cannot avoid overall accountability for the actions of those responsible.

The ability of a leader to effectively delegate authority while maintaining accountability is limited to a manageable span of control. Span of control describes how many people one person can personally supervise successfully. Depending on the source one cites, the accepted number is between three and seven people, with five being the optimal number. This is important for leaders to keep in mind when a preplanning project becomes large or involves multiple parts. Working within the effective span of control helps ensure that necessary tasks will be completed and will not get "lost" in the process.

## Training

Training levels must be viewed from a financial standpoint as well as from a technological perspective. By taking into consideration the current funding and available technology, EMS agencies can assess how they will be able to complete the preplanning process for a particular event, incident, or facility.

Training should be tied in with the preplanning process whenever possible, because it prepares responders for dealing with multiple projected scenarios and provides a practical evaluation of a standard procedure. If, during a training session, an EMS agency discovers that a certain aspect of operations is impractical, this information can be used to modify the preplan. Training is also important for incident preplanning, because it familiarizes crews and command with new personnel, equipment, and technology. It can be used to introduce and put into practice any modifications to ERPs. Training is necessary for individual personnel, crews, and management, as well as receiving and sending facilities integrated into an agency preplan. Four types of training are typically used in EMS: classroom (cognitive and psychomotor), drills (psychomotor and affective), tabletop, and exercises.

In a classroom setting, an instructor who is a subject matter expert will present a set of expectations or objectives to the class, outlining the goals of the training. Personnel are then guided through various tasks designed to increase their knowledge base. They are graded based on a set of criteria, which has been developed by both the instructor and the organization to meet the recognized standards. Drills test EMS personnel's ability to recall and implement standard procedure by asking crews to respond to simulated scenarios. Drills are done by individual personnel, crews, shifts, an entire EMS agency, or multiple coordinating EMS agencies. Tabletop exercises are meant for management, providers, and primary response agencies. Exercises help to test the capability of an organization to respond to a simulated event. The exercise tests multiple functions of an organization's operational plan, and is a coordinated response to a situation in a time-pressured, realistic simulation that involves several agencies. It focuses on the coordination, integration, and interaction of an organization's policies, procedures, roles, and responsibilities before, during, or after the simulated event. It places heavy emphasis on communication between all the agencies participating in the exercise.

Individual training objectives should be obtainable, realistic, and reproducible. Each objective should be regarded as a core competency, based on a specific standard or the requirements of a preplan, outlining the level of performance required of an agency's responders. These core competencies must apply to individuals, crews, the agency overall, and should guide coordination with outside agencies. Collective objectives of training should encompass multiple tasks—interrelated because of their use in a given response scenario—that will be required of personnel.

Incorporation of training evaluation into preplan development fulfills the planning cycle of: plan, act, do, and evaluate. To make preplanning effective, training and evaluation of personnel and procedure should be ongoing processes. The benefits of training are lost if it is done infrequently. Training should also be modified in response to significant changes in key personnel, major equipment, and technology.

## Availability of Equipment

Another issue encountered when dealing with personnel is the selection and distribution of proper personal protective equipment (PPE). It is important for preplanning administration to assess whether there is enough of the right type(s) of PPE available in the proper sizes. In order to meet the unique needs of a team, more equipment may need to be purchased. PPE may also require additional or recurring training, such as annual fit testing of masks. Certain equipment might mandate physicals, such as in a hazardous materials team, prior to being able to use the equipment. It is essential that as agencies take on additional capability, the administration also assumes and understands its responsibility for providing the necessary resources, training, and physicals to keep team members safe during a response. One secondary issue that is assumed with planning responses for hazardous materials, for instance, is the need for immunizations that may be required for personnel using certain kinds of protective equipment.

# Resources

Before beginning the preplanning process, it is important to assess what is needed to get the project done. First, it is necessary to examine internal resources. All agencies have resources, such as information technology (IT), management information system (MIS), or the local lexicon for computers and associated communication mechanisms. If the agency is fire-based, they will also have access to past fire plans and inspections. Likewise, if any of the previously mentioned items are not internally available to the agency responsible for preplanning, it is considered an external resource.

Externally, an EMS agency can look to emergency management, state, regional, and federal assets as resources. When a city is selected for the Super Bowl, for instance, many additional state and federal resources are made available for planning and integration purposes. The closer it gets to the playoff date, the more resources are fed into the local processes for planning and response.

External resources could also come from other fire departments or EMS agencies, including other city or municipal departments involved in preplanning. The parks department, for example, may have a plan for a specific facility or may allow for utilization of certain resources, such as water from local swimming pools, in the case of a fire. The water department may also have plans or resources available to agencies engaged in the preplanning process. Other external resources may come from unlikely people such as vendors, who may have inventory support available or may even be able to make contacts between different agencies, following a template appropriate for a particular type of event. Wherever external support can be found, it is important to explore those options and evaluate their potential.

Additional external resources may include administrative bodies. These can be legal bodies, foundations, or private organizations that may be willing to help the preplanning effort. Certain private entities will be willing to support preplanning possibilities if an agency's request is phrased the right way.

Resources require budgets in some form or another. Resource-related expenses fall under an agency's budget or sub-budget. Besides direct resources required for preplanning, there are also indirect or shared resources that must be addressed in the work processes. Sharing resources can produce a choke point or potential roadblock in the preplanning effort, as the resource is not guaranteed to be available when it is needed. An agency will need to coordinate with whoever is responsible for the desired resource before incorporating it into its preplan. This is a good example of why an administration advocate is needed to protect the preplanning process.

Another resource that is overlooked by those "in the trenches" is the budget. Many "trench-level" people will be needed to examine whether the budget is sufficient, because it will affect a future incident outcome. These frontline personnel will know best what the repercussions will be of having an inadequate amount of a particular resource. The budget is also important because whoever controls the budget will also control the preplanning workflow. In this way, the budget serves an administrative function, dictating how preplanning should proceed. Hazard vulnerability analyses (HVA) needs to be performed and gap analyses must be conducted, in order to determine an initial budgetary estimate. Through completion of an HVA, preplanners can recognize specific hazards and consider any required equipment that may have an impact on the budget. Gap analyses will identify whether additional equipment needs to be purchased, trained, or even considered. The administrative function of the budget kicks in once a decision is made to purchase or acquire certain resources, equipment, personnel, or training. The next step is to determine where in the budget these funds for additional equipment and training will come from. It is then necessary to determine whether these new items will be capital items, ordered with a purchase card, or acquired through a purchase order.

## Current Administrative Posture

In preparation for preplanning, or in its beginning stages, it is important for an organization to evaluate where it stands, from an administrative perspective. A good place to begin such an evaluation is with a consideration of the organization's administrative foundation, which describes a particular agency's directives, policies, and guidelines. These are what drive the organization on a daily basis. An EMS agency's policies reflect the team's guiding principles and values. It is also important to identify which of the current policies, directions, or directives will be affected by the preplanning process. Preplanning may modify or completely eliminate an agency's standard procedure. An old plan may not adequately meet current emergency response needs. A preplanning effort will address new technologies and methods that will improve an agency's ability to serve the region it is responsible for protecting.

## Unexpected Consequences

Primary and secondary effects of an emergency incident must be considered when preplanning. The unpredictable nature of an incident scene mandates an evaluation of how agency resources will be impacted by secondary incident effects. The other aspect of this is examining how unexpected changes at an incident scene will impact an agency's ability to respond to further issues that come to the fore. The purchase of new equipment for a disaster or special event, for instance, may cost an organization $1,000. If this purchase significantly changes the way an organization operates on emergency scenes, it may either increase or decrease further operational issues and capabilities. Consider the example of purchasing a large mass-treatment tent for use during large outdoor festivities: While this purchase may be justified and utilized throughout its useful life, if this item is not anticipated within the current budget, the purchase of other items in the budget may need to be postponed. Preplanning with these potential changes in mind can prepare an organization to adequately and cost-effectively respond to the ever-evolving incident scene.

# Documentation

It is said that a job is not done until the paperwork is done. Documentation begins before an incident occurs; the preplanning effort for a particular incident or event must be documented. Many postincident processes will depend on complete documentation. For example, when federal reimbursement is requested for certain items purchased with a grant, there must be documentation confirming that the purchase was made. There must also be documentation, such as photographs of the old equipment, proving what condition the item was in before an incident.

The preplanning process also must be documented. A record must be kept of meeting notes, plan modification, and incident or event research. Preincident documentation is used by agencies to reduce liability issues after the incident. The planning process proves that the organization worked with due diligence and to the best of its ability, within the scope of its mission, with access to a given set of resources. This will assist if there is a question of "Well, did you consider this, did you do that?" It is documented that an organization did make these considerations during preplanning. In terms of liability, it is better to have a flawed plan documented than to have no plan at all. Many agencies and government bodies will take minutes of meetings so that they can address any concerns as to what was discussed or worked on, as well as potential problems, or consequences to not acting in a given situation.

## Documentation of Equipment

Documenting equipment is essential for accountability, just as fire departments and EMS agencies must document after large fires or crashes. Accounting for the use of high-value items, such as cardiac monitors and ventilators, is part of the job. EMS agencies must keep records, to determine whether replacement parts need to be bought or equipment needs servicing after use. Some of these concerns may be in relation to capital budget items (for certain agencies, over $10,000 is allotted). It is possible, however, that an EMS agency could respond to a hazardous material incident where a cardiac monitor was contaminated. The monitor may have to be thrown away and may have constituted an expense of $10,000 to $20,000. This is a significant amount of money for many departments, and in order to gain replacement funds, documentation showing what occurred and why certain things happened is important.

## Documentation of Training

Training must also be documented. Administration must have a record of the base level of training its responders have received. It must also know the base level of training required for its personnel, given the tasks regularly performed by the agency. Documenting personnel physicals is also a crucial administrative task. EMS agencies must keep records stating that physicals were administered properly, by certified physicians. If regional standards state that all employees charged with a certain task must have a specific blood mercury level—a common requirement for hazardous materials scenes—then it needs to be documented when and by whom the appropriate physical was performed.

## Documentation of Meetings and Coordination

Meetings with outside agencies, departments, or entities—especially private ones—also merit documentation. It is important to document persons who have been contacted along with the result of that contact. Once again, this may lessen liability, but it also validates the preplanning effort. Items to address with the documentation may vary for different organizations, based upon state laws, where financing comes from, and whether there are relevant legal issues within a particular community. It is important to document the dates as well as the duration of these meetings, to verify that a certain preplanning goal was accomplished in the course of the meeting.

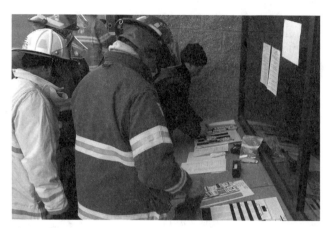

**Figure 11-3** It is imperative that EMS personnel document all incident response activities. This includes keeping accurate and thorough records of patient care.

## Document Operations

Although this section concerns administration, it is also important to mention that operational incidents must be documented as well. It is a good idea to document what was done on, around, or near an incident or facility if something unexpected occurs on scene (see **Figure 11-3**). Such documentation would be managed by the finance or logistics section of ICS. Emergency responders must ensure that a log of critical events is maintained, so that an organization may be able to defend its proceedings or accurately recount events when faced with liability issues. The log should identify persons assigned to each function established at an incident scene, especially key functions. Who, for instance, served as the operations section chief? The log must be presented in a format that is easy to use for on-scene personnel. It should also organize information in a clear manner, so that the postincident analysis team may use it to reconstruct the events of the incident.

Basic items within the log might include the names of personnel assigned to specific functions, when those personnel accomplished their given tasks, the point at which command was assumed, details concerning staffing, the names of those who responded via mutual aid requests, and when they were called to the scene.

## Postincident Documentation

There is a definite need to document a few things after the incident. One of the key things is the after action report (AAR) or critique. The AAR, the postincident critique, or training done in response to a postincident analysis are important because they provide documentation that a postincident review was completed and is key to maintaining federal monies, as well as having the ability to get more training and equipment later on. The AAR can also identify what part of the plan(s) did not work or which part of the plans worked but was impractical.

# Fulfilling the Needs of EMS Personnel

This section addresses the three "Ms" of personnel needs: medical, mental health, and monetary needs. The first "M" that the organization should provide are the appropriate medical care/ examinations to be performed before and after incidents. An example is if there is a hazardous materials incident, there should be some sort of an examination after the fact to ensure that the personnel who responded do not have any issues upon conclusion of the incident.

The next "M," mental, is having people screened informally, not forcibly, for mental issues, both temporary and longer term, such as post-traumatic stress disorder (PTSD). Is there some sort of method that mandates or at least asks the question 6 months after a "significant incident," so the agency can identify how people are doing? What is going on in their lives; maybe there is an increase in divorce or suicide? What about sick leave utilization or incidents of on-the-job alcohol use? Those items are particularly important to document, not so much to cast blame,

### Preplanning Practices

If EMS must deviate from protocols because of unusual circumstances, responders should consult with online medical control and make sure they document it well on their patient care reports.

but to identify so that employees can get the help that they need. This is taking care of the employees as people.

Next, there are monetary issues: Was there a hazardous materials incident that caused personnel to stay past their shift change for 3 hours? Did everyone get paid for it? If so, who was on standby? Are there rules in the state, the city, or municipality with agreements that state if someone was on standby, they need to get paid?

It is important to remember that the job does not end after the incident is mitigated. EMS needs to remember to care for its employees. Remembering the three "Ms" can promote unity and a family environment.

> **Preplanning Practices**
>
> The primary needs of emergency care providers fall into three categories, known as the three "Ms:"
>
> Medical examinations
> Mental well-being assessment
> Monetary compensation

## Selected References

Covey, SR: *Leadership: Great Leaders, Great Teams, Great Results*, audio CD. Salt Lake City, UT: Franklin Covey Company; 2007.

George, ML: *Lean Six Sigma for Service*. New York, NY: The McGraw-Hill Companies; 2003.

Hutton, DW: *The Change Agent's Handbook*. Milwaukee, WI: ASQ Quality Press; 1994.

International City/County Management Association: *Managing Fire and Rescue Services*. Washington, D.C.: ICMA Press; 2002.

International City/County Management Association: *Managing Fire Services*, 2nd ed. Washington, D.C.: ICMA Press; 1988.

Kramer, WM and Bahme, CW: *Fire Officer's Guide to Disaster Control*. 2nd ed. Saddle Brook, NJ: Fire Engineering Books and Videos, Penwell Publishing; 1992.

Smith, JP *Strategic and Tactical Considerations on the Fireground*. Upper Saddle River, NJ: Brady Books, Pearson; 2002.

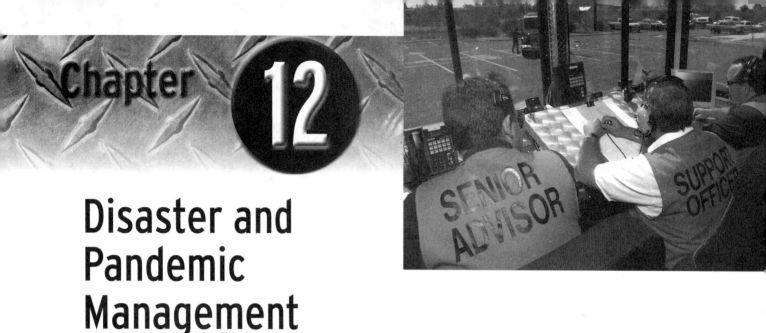

# Chapter 12

# Disaster and Pandemic Management

## Planning for the Unimaginable

In the Army there is a motto that says, "Train like you fight and fight like you train." This means people will respond and react to circumstances as they have trained. Therefore, good training leads to effective operations. Emergency medical services (EMS) personnel function in a similar emergency setting that requires them to respond to incidents with which they may or may not be familiar, such as a possible terrorist attack involving over 500 poisoned patients. The Army motto can be carried over to EMS and fire services. Throughout the duration of an incident, conditions change and new obstacles develop. This characteristic of emergency incidents requires EMS responders to have strong training that allows them to think on their feet and provide quality patient care. It is especially important for EMS agencies to implement preplans in preparation for major disasters so that responders will have direction even under uncertain and dangerous circumstances.

The Army trains for worldwide deployments with variable factors such as terrain, population density, and capability of potential enemies. In doing so, they develop and use a common task list. This technique can also carry over well into EMS response. The military term for this list is mission essential task list (METL). While EMS does not rely on a METL per se, EMS organizations can and should develop a checklist or emergency response plan (ERP) outlining the basic tasks that need to be carried out. This checklist should be based on findings from the hazard vulnerability analysis (HVA) (see chapter 4). This list needs to be created at all levels regardless of any variables, such as supply or staffing shortages, that need to be addressed in order for a crew to accomplish its mission.

A common key element between the METL and an EMS task list is that all lower elements and functions associated with a response must fit into the next higher echelon of command. Every component must fit into the overall mission goal. Whether looking at the task from the top to bottom or vice versa, the tasks must be integrated so that each step is fully supported. It is especially important to have a working task list when responding to weapons of mass destruction (WMD), hazardous materials, pandemics, and severe acute respiratory syndrome (SARS) type calls, as these are not incidents EMS responds to on a day-to-day basis. Having a list of what needs to be accomplished is an effective preplanning tool, because it allows EMS agencies to balance what they are currently doing and what they are planning to do against what they know needs to be accomplished in preparation for a disaster or pandemic. The checklist for a chemical spill may include items such as:

1. Contacting the local emergency departments and advising them of the potential to receive contaminated patients coming in via private auto.
2. Minimizing the amount of ambulances transporting contaminated patients by designating specific ambulances to transport patients.
3. Ensuring an adequate number of personnel has been recalled from off-duty to assist in the incident.

## Applying the 80/20 Rule

A comprehensive task list allows EMS agencies to plan for 80% of what can be expected during a response to a given incident. This is known as the 80/20 rule (see chapter 3). This same rule is used in federal planning and training. Agencies should look to the Department of Transportation (DOT) *Emergency Response Guidebook (ERG)* to research common elements of particular incidents. Approximately 80% of management for each particular type of disaster or pandemic has common concerns. Common methods of dispatch, response, support, and communications are used to manage each of these incidents. When agencies plan for events such as WMD, SARS, or pandemic influenza, they need to first consider the 80% of characteristics that are common to the all incidents, and then they can begin to deal with the 20% that are variables: When evaluating the 20% of the management that is variable, 80% of it is common to similar types of incidents. So, for example, 80% of the management of a hazardous materials incident is the same for a pandemic. In the 20% of variable management in a hazardous materials incident, 80% of that is the same whether it is a chemical, radiological, or biologic incident.

## Considering Lessons Learned

A common lesson learned in dealing with events worldwide has been that operational failure often is linked to weakness in communications. In the experience of EMS and other emergency response agencies, this has been a result of the technological failure of communications systems as well as the failure of personnel to properly use the communications systems that were already in place. The lack of a functional information management system tends to correlate with inadequate communications and management system training. Following Hurricane Katrina, the US Conference of Mayors sponsored a survey that found that 60% of cities involved in the emergency response experienced a failure of communications systems, preventing their police and fire radios from contacting state emergency operations centers (EOCs). Ninety-seven percent of cities with major chemical plants were unable to communicate with the plant's security force. The survey also cited incompatibility between 80% of city emergency networks with federal communications systems.

Multiple plans and guidelines are needed to ensure that communications failures do not lead to inefficient emergency response. Experience has shown that a lack of written plans and guidelines will slow the notification and response of proper authorities. Responders

### Preplanning Practices

Overall, it is important to keep plans simple. Disasters and pandemics are complicated incidents. Plans that are too complicated, based on multiple variables, will fail. Agencies must make sure that what responders are being asked to do is simple in writing as well as in execution, because disasters and pandemics are not events that happen all the time. EMS agencies need to consider the normal responding crews' ability to do their daily job and then proceed with the development of the preplan.

should be discouraged from operating based on their own memory of such protocol. Agencies should provide communications procedures in a written format so that when responders need to implement the plan, they can refer to a physical document. Just as a checklist is invaluable to agency preplanners, especially for unexpected incidents, accessible and tangible response protocols leave less room for error at an incident response.

## Assessing Capabilities

Before defining the roles and responsibilities of individual responders (to be incorporated into an METL), EMS agencies need to conduct an assessment of their capabilities:

- What resources (eg, personnel, equipment, supplies) are available at the incident scene?
- How proficient and competent are an agency's responders in certain aspects of emergency response? What areas are they less experienced in?
- Who is capable of accomplishing each necessary response task?

EMS agencies should have primary and secondary plans in place to ensure functions get taken care of, such as decontamination. If decontamination is needed, it is important to have redundancy in place in anticipation of the event that a particular response unit, such as a hazardous materials unit, is busy, injured, or taken out of service (such as during 9/11 attacks at the World Trade Center). This will allow a backup plan, which can be put in place rapidly to replace lost or out-of-service assets.

It is likely that multiple agencies will be called upon to respond to a natural disaster, act of terrorism, or widespread pandemic. EMS also must assess where their response activities overlap with these other agencies' efforts:

- What are these points of overlap?
- If needed, what agreement must be established between agencies to coordinate response efforts?

## Exercising Empathy

Finally, although response agencies make plans for multiple potential incidents, it is important to understand that their personnel will be dealing with people. These people may be afraid, contaminated, or dealing with other personal issues and pre-existing medical conditions. The purpose of an act of terrorism is to inflict terror and to make people afraid to live as they did prior to the incident. Emergency care providers must be very cognizant of this, so that they do not enhance the terror aspect by becoming afraid and panicked themselves or by being too callous in their actions. Such behavior will cause EMS to frighten the very people they are trying to protect.

# Common Elements of WMD Incidents

When preplanning for incidents involving WMD, it is important to define the term as specifically as possible. The acronym CBRNE goes into further detail: chemical, biological, radiological, nuclear, and explosive. This chapter will use the abbreviation, WMD, but in doing so will refer all of the terms detailed in CBRNE. In the general sense, a WMD event is one that is designed to overwhelm local resources, create a single or multiple catastrophic events, overwhelm emergency responders and the response mechanism, and produce multiple injuries.

National Fire Protection Association (NFPA) Standard 472, *Standard for Competence of Responders to Hazardous Materials/Weapons of Mass Destruction Incidents*, defines hazardous material as: "A substance (either matter—solid, liquid, or gas—or energy) that when released is capable of creating harm to people, the environment, and property, including weapons of mass destruction (WMD) as defined in 18 US Code, Section 2332a, as well as any other criminal use of hazardous materials, such as illicit labs, environmental crimes, or industrial sabotage." A common characteristic of WMD events is the use of hazardous materials.

A chemical spill may be planned or accidental. Emergency response plans should be developed based on established protocol for dealing with hazardous chemical releases (refer to the *ERG* for guidance on responses to specific chemicals). Biological warfare describes the planned release of a biological toxin or agent to create fear or inflict multiple casualties on a city, municipality, or state. Radiological agents are materials that emit radioactivity (the spontaneous decay or disintegration of an unstable atomic nucleus accompanied by emission of radiation) and can be dispersed in an effort to contaminate an area with radioactive materials. A nuclear threat could involve the presence of an explosive device that uses fusion, fission, or both to cause mass destruction. Explosive devices also depend on the combustive reactions of their hazardous components and can be used to inflict widespread terror and injury. Bombings are the most frequent terrorist acts.

In the case of a pandemic, EMS personnel usually think about pandemic influenza. A pandemic describes the spread of a virus that affects a very large region; patient symptoms and geographical area must be taken into consideration when preplanning for pandemics. The 1918 pandemic influenza claimed the lives of 20 to 50 million people worldwide. This and subsequent influenza pandemics were caused by new strains of the human flu virus that spread rapidly, because people had not yet developed immunity to it. The flu cannot be prevented by vaccinations alone. The single most important thing that EMS organizations can do to help in the face of pandemic influenza is to utilize good hand hygiene and contact precautions to help in minimizing the spread of infectious agents.

SARS is a virus that is resistant to treatment. The 2003 outbreak of SARS in Toronto, Canada had a profound impact on EMS in that city. Refer to the following case study.

| CBRNE |
|---|
| WMD may refer to any of the following: <br><br> Chemical <br> Biological <br> Radiological <br> Nuclear <br> Explosive |

## Case Study

Toronto EMS felt SARS' impact when it experienced 1,116 potential SARS exposures in 850 paramedics. Regarded as one of the largest and most active municipal EMS organizations in Canada, it transports over 140,000 patients to 17 different hospitals annually. During the SARS outbreak, however, of the organization's potential exposures, 436 paramedics required 10-day home quarantine. With an incubation period of more than a week, the potential for cross-contamination of patients remained an ominous possibility. In order for Toronto EMS to maintain continuity of care, all personnel had to be screened for SARS-like symptoms prior to assisting with response operations. Personnel presenting with such symptoms reported to the medical unit and withdrew from the EMS response effort.

Through their experience with the 2003 SARS pandemic, Toronto EMS learned the importance of implementing an emergency plan prior to a potential pandemic outbreak. They also found that it was essential to establish rapid and functional methods of communication with provincial and municipal

*continues*

health authorities, to ensure the availability of the most up-to-date outbreak information. To facilitate this, intergovernment relationships could be established in advance. Furthermore, the fears of frontline personnel can also be managed effectively with timely and accurate communication. Until the risk of exposure was considered negligible, Toronto EMS learned the value of maintaining personal protective equipment (PPE) procedures.

# Responding to WMD Incidents

The difference between incidents lies in how fast they happen and the expected duration of the responses to each disaster. In general, WMD incidents are fast-acting events. They happen either intentionally or unintentionally and are usually quite rapid in the expansion, toxicity, or lethality of the event. A chemical attack is a purposeful act, whereas as a hazardous materials release is usually accidental. The effect is the same, because whatever chemical is present, it is hazardous to people, and the rate of spread is based on variables such as temperature, wind, sun, and chemical properties of the agent involved. On the other hand, biological incidents such pandemic flu and SARS are relatively slow-progressing incidents. They usually happen over a period of a few days, and EMS is able to see the warning signs. Because biological disasters are not part of day-to-day operations, however, EMS agencies often miss the warning signs that a biological incident is taking place. It is important for EMS to establish and foster a good working relationship with either the local public health agency or the infectious disease physicians at the local hospital(s) for warning and notification of biological events.

How do EMS agencies prepare, detect, and respond to a WMD incident? According to a 2007 study by Scot Phelps, only 4% of the Department of Homeland Security (DHS) funding for public safety terrorism was allotted to EMS. The main reason for having DHS funding is to provide a means for facilitating responses to multiple incidents. The vast majority of the DHS budget goes to police, then to fire agencies, and finally to EMS. Because of the lack of federal funding for EMS organizations, typically budgets overlook WMD preparation, events are deemphasized, and response is ill-prepared.

In terms of detection and response for hazardous materials incidents, how are response agencies notified that one has occurred? Usually, someone will make a 9-1-1 call saying that a spill, crash, or train derailment has taken place. Sensors at facilities may have also gone off to signal the hazardous event. Usually, the response is point-specific, and EMS agencies will travel to one geographical location, identify the hazard, and proceed accordingly. Hazardous materials incidents are normal responses for most EMS and fire agencies. It is an everyday concept; many agencies run hazardous materials drills on a weekly or monthly basis, in an attempt to train for the expected hazards.

## Chemical and Radiological Incident Detection

Chemical or radiological events usually occur at a specific site, and area-specific sensors may go off. People nearby may hear a big bang, or responding agencies may find a lot of people who are dead or dying in one particular area. A plane may have flown overhead, for instance, and dropped what appeared to be crop-dusting chemicals. The event of a chemical or radiological release is usually an obvious event. Phelps' study also showed that in the event of a chemical release, 44 out of 50 or 88 percent of EMS systems did not have the capability to support decontamination procedures. Responding to a chemical or radiological incident requires the use of hazardous materials suits or other PPE. Level A hazardous materials suits are typically needed on events such as these. There are various requirements, however, that preclude a responder's utilization of such PPE. Responders must complete training on operations inside of a Level A suit and must have some prior experience operating in an enclosed environment with an increased ambient temperature (see **Figure 12-1**). The bunker gear worn by firefighters and some EMS personnel may not be suitable for dealing with a chemical environment, depending on what agent has been released.

## Biological Incident Detection

Bioterrorism events can be widespread incidents. Calls may come through 9-1-1, but notification and detection may also come through emergency departments or by trend reports from the public health officer. As a result, the location and nature of the incident may not immediately be obvious. EMS may be still running multiple calls for respiratory and cardiac emergencies, as they do every other day, and not realize that they are slowly increasing in the amount of respiratory or other issues. EMS may just see a spike in service delivery calls—maybe a 10 percent to 15 percent increase in call volume—and so it may be difficult for EMS to respond to a biological incident right away. A unique characteristic of biological agents, and even pandemic flu to a certain extent, is that emergency responders could expect exponential growth. Large amounts of people in one geographical area will start to present with similar signs and symptoms.

Pandemic influenza and SARS also will impact a wide area. Most detection goes through the emergency rooms as well as some public health determinants. Some of the indicators that public health may be able to tell us are available through school or other reporting mechanisms. The public health department can use these resources to identify what is going on. Once again, pandemics and SARS exhibit exponential growth, as infected persons continue to infect others. An infected person, for instance, has the ability to infect three others, resulting in the accelerated spread of illness.

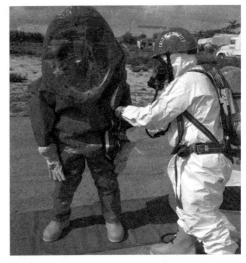

**Figure 12-1** Before participating in emergency response for hazardous materials incidents, EMS personnel must be properly trained in the use of the appropriate PPE.

# Coordination for Disasters and Pandemics

As with all preplanning, an EMS agency's preparation for responses to disasters and pandemics begins with coordination of resources and responses with the following entities: hospitals, public health, law enforcement, logistics, hazardous materials or fire departments, administration, training, nongovernment organizations (NGOs), and public information officers (PIOs).

## Hospitals

Hospitals may be points of detection, decontamination, triage, treatment, and recovery. Hospitals are community assets that need to be identified, secured, maintained, and utilized properly. When coordinating with hospitals, EMS agencies should look into alternative care sites and set those up in preparation for potential incidents. EMS organizations must ask the following questions: Will an alternative care site need to be set up? If so, where should it be located (eg, a local school gym)? What procedures should be followed to ensure that it is stocked throughout the duration of the emergency response? Although these issues are typically handled by the hospital, it is important for EMS to understand. Also, EMS agencies will need to consider the command structure at a given hospital: Who will be in charge? How will the hospital handle a surge? Can the staff deal with it? Will the hospital have intensive care unit (ICU) beds? What is its surge capability and how long can it be sustained? Having this information is vital in order for EMS agencies to adequately incorporate hospitals into their preplans for disasters and pandemics.

## Public Health

Public health is also a function of detection, decontamination, community response, triage, and treatment. Part of their job is syndromic surveillance, which means they keep an eye on the overall health and wellness within the community. Part of the function of public health is detection and making appropriate notifications: How does public health coordinate with regional response? What is their state and federal notification procedure? Will they notify EMS when a notification procedure is established or modified? Where does EMS fall on the tree for notification, and who is going to make that notification? EMS must ascertain those elements of public health's responsibilities during a disaster or pandemic. Agencies should have no doubt public health will do its job, but should investigate where EMS falls within its standard protocol.

## Law Enforcement

EMS agencies must coordinate the security of individual or multiple incident sites, depending on the scale of the incident. Coordinating with law enforcement during preplanning for disasters and pandemics includes asking the question: Where are the responders going to be? This information should be provided to law enforcement, so that law enforcement personnel can oversee operations from a safety standpoint. EMS organizations need to assess the security of the storage facilities and distribution facilities if medications are going to be given to the public. This information is also imperative for the police to understand.

If victims are given clear instructions, they will fare well as a majority. There are times, however, when people are not given instructions. When emergency responders leave incident victims to their own devices, this is when chaos ensues. Once chaos takes hold, it is very hard for responders to regain control of a scene. To protect the logistics branch, hospital personnel, and EMS personnel who are interacting with patients must know what law enforcement's plans are to provide security. Responders also need to understand limitations of this safety plan and, if a limitation is reached, how personnel will be notified when the safety protocol has reached its limit without overwhelming the people impacted by the incident, resulting in a surge where victims could potentially hurt responders.

The other function of law enforcement is to provide civil peace at the scene of an incident. During EMS preplanning, organizations should ask law enforcement the following questions: What is the police's plan for providing civil peace? Are enough officers available to provide adequate security for responders, incident sites, and security as EMS performs its normal every-day functions? One fear is that, in the event of a biological incident such as SARS or pandemic flu, people will have difficulty accessing the emergency room and physicians. This will lead to an increase in 9-1-1 calls. If these calls create a backup in EMS operations, it will put crews at increased risk for responding to normal calls.

## Logistics and Support

In coordinating with logistics and support, EMS agencies must ask: Will there be a need for specialized equipment? For a chemical response, one should assume that such equipment is necessary. For a pandemic influenza response, there might not be a similar need, because the response requires normal equipment that is already utilized on a day-to-day basis. After this question has been answered, EMS organizations must track the availability of any specialized equipment, antidotes, masks, or basic IV fluids—essentially, basic supplies needed to provide emergency care. If EMS runs a larger amount of calls than usual, it is important for them to determine the following, jointly with logistics: How can a vendor be secured that is able to rapidly provide EMS with the items it needs?

Transportation issues that should be preplanned in cooperation with logistics include ensuring that fuel is available for transportation. For example, if an event occurs where a local community hospital has been temporarily shut down because it is overwhelmed or perhaps an EMS agency is called to the site of a hazardous materials spill, there must be enough fuel to transport personnel, equipment, and supplies to where they are needed. If the plan calls for EMS to divert past a local hospital, go to another hospital, or travel to another region, are maps or global positioning systems (GPS) available to show these routes? What contact information is available, that EMS may use to let other responders know what is going on?

Finally, if an incident turns out to be a long-term issue, EMS agencies must organize support for the provision of food and water to crews as they deal with the emergency. Preplanning for the extended duration of a disaster or pandemic may involve setting up a rehabilitation sector. EMS organizations need to be aware of these long-term plans, so that on-scene personnel will be prepared to modify operations as the incident evolves.

## Hazardous Materials Teams

In terms of hazardous materials teams, EMS agencies must understand what their capabilities are, what they are not capable of, where they can operate from, and what is needed to support them. The general responsibilities for a hazardous materials team are detection, decontamination, runoff containment of the event. Depending on the capabilities of the agency, it may be the hazardous materials team's function or a state function to come in later and prevent a secondary site contamination such as runoff. EMS agencies need to coordinate, if the fire department is not in their home agency, how the outside fire department will notify EMS about a hazardous materials incident. It is also important, during preplanning, for EMS agencies to answer the following questions: How will the hazardous materials team respond? Who will be in charge of patient triage and treatment? Will these tasks be an EMS function, or will they be a fire department function?

## Administration

EMS needs to understand the EMS administration of standard operations procedures (SOPs), standard operating guidelines (SOGs), directives, rules, and regulations. This involves having administrative plans for such tasks as recall, staffing, and requesting mutual aid. Administration may also need to coordinate for a legal provision, such as state law or federal law requiring physicals, or for other legal issues that need to be addressed and outlined in writing to comply with Occupational Safety and Health Administration (OSHA), Superfund Amendments and Reauthorization Act (SARA), and other federal and state regulations. Records must be maintained, and administration must ensure records are available to be filled out immediately.

A key area for consideration during preplanning for disasters or pandemics is staffing. The Canadian experience with SARS showed that approximately one third of nurses in hospitals did not report for duty either out of fear of the infection or because of family concerns such as sick family members. In planning for long-term staffing, it is important to have measures for relief of those already on duty and for the security and safety of responder families. Many communities have heeded this lesson from the Canadian SARS response and now include immediate family members in any immunization or prophylactic care given to responders. This allows EMS to alleviate the staff's fears for what may happen to their families.

## Training

Oftentimes overlooked, training needs to be coordinated prior to disaster. Training deals with individual training, crew training, and department training. It should cover the most recent standards and laws such as NFPA Standards 471 through 473, the OSHA laws, and the Code of Federal Regulations (CFR) 1910 series that deal with hazardous materials incidents. When preparing for a response to a specific incident, EMS staff can go back to the emergency response plan (ERP) and evaluate what the team's capabilities are. Once this evaluation is complete, EMS teams can begin to train with their strengths and weaknesses in mind. Training for disasters and pandemics includes training administrative staff, clerical workers, people tasked with housekeeping, and ancillary personnel. Preincident training ensures that everyone will understand what their roles are and allows EMS agencies to plan for the most appropriate use of its human resources.

Many medical facilities use "paper drills" in preparation for major disasters. This involves outlining a preplanned response on a piece of paper, then walking all involved personnel through the process. This kind of drill works well for most clinical responders, but can become an issue for nonclinical personnel in hospitals. Most agencies will not incorporate logistics personnel in operational drills. As with practicing for a cardiac arrest or "code," unless EMS agencies practice all the involved elements, responders are going to forget the small but often critical things. Sometimes the small oversights end up hurting someone on scene. Understanding training's role in preplanning for disasters and pandemics, as a result, is especially important.

## Nongovernment Organizations

NGOs include supportive organizations and other municipal departments. These organizations include the American Red Cross, Salvation Army, citizens fire academy, and citizens police academy. These organizations are there to support the response, the victims, and the responders. EMS agencies need to understand what these organizations' support functions are, what they can provide, when can they provide it, and what their limitations are.

Understanding the limitations of nongovernment assistance is a critical preplanning task. Many people, out of the goodness of their hearts, will offer many response functions in the time of an emergency. It is sometimes the case, however, that they do not have enough people trained or that their personnel are physically or mentally exhausted and cannot perform.

Support functions of NGOs may include the provision of heavy equipment such as a contractor. Depending on the incident and the organization, provision of heavy equipment may be deemed a command function. Many times, however, EMS agencies limit themselves to just dealing with patients. Nevertheless, it is important that EMS agencies be aware of local, available rescue organizations that will have expertise to supplement the actual providers' efforts on scene. NGOs might be able to help with extrication, for example, or provide other functions that are missing from the response plan.

## Public Information Officer

Many times EMS organizations forget about the function and responsibilities of the media. All EMS personnel must realize, however, that when a terrorist event such as a WMD attack occurs, that information has to be given to the public, and it is essential that there be one clear message given. It is not reassuring for the public to hear five different messages coming from five different response agencies. As a result, EMS needs to coordinate and work with the PIO, understanding who will be designated PIO for certain events, and determine what agency will have an established PIO function, so that the coordinating agencies can cohesively address questions from the press.

It is possible for EMS organizations to provide resources to the PIO on how to respond to questions. PIOs have many different modes of communication available to them. The PIO may choose to address public concerns via the Internet. Regardless of the medium it is transmitted on, however, it is essential that one consistent message is provided to the public. EMS does not have the luxury of waiting for print to come out the next day. EMS agencies must release a unified message to the public. The public will evaluate EMS actions based on the message.

## Ongoing Operations

The occurrence of WMD incidents will have an impact on 9-1-1 calls. Depending on the type of event, 9-1-1 usage may actually decrease as on September 11, 2001, during the initial impact as people understood what was happening. In such a case, responses to calls concerning more common emergencies will decrease slightly as time goes on. There will still be a need to respond to chest pains, respiratory emergencies such as asthma, and diabetic calls. These types of calls will not wait for the resolution of a disaster. As a result, EMS must plan for continuity of care. This may be accomplished through a mutual aid agreement (MAA) or through private contractors, being contracted to a 9-1-1 or mutual aid response. Despite the needs of a major disaster, EMS agencies will still be running most of their regular calls. In the event of a major disaster, it is often the case that one incident is prompting multiple people to call. It will be important for EMS to work and communicate with dispatchers, so that dispatchers can filter through many calls to realize they are not regarding many separate incidents (see **Figure 12-2**).

Biologic, pandemic, and SARS incidents may entail a relatively gradual increase in response needs. While EMS may already be responding, it is possible that they have not figured out what they are responding to as they are going along. EMS needs to be aware that while the increase in calls may be gradual, it may also be depleting agencies' strength and resources.

Major disasters will take a toll on EMS standard of care. In EMS, as in any medical operation, standard of care is important. It is a set of principles saying what an agency will do to provide care for the patients they come in contact with. It is usually an immovable standard for the majority of cases: An agency will ensure, for instance, that people with chest pains will get 12-leads. People who need to go to the catheter lab will get there. Diabetics will get dextrose. People with traumatic injuries will be taken to the operating room. During a disaster, alteration in care is something EMS organizations must address and possibly incorporate. Issues relating to standard of care include EMS staffing, response processes, units in service, alternative destinations, Health Insurance Portability and Accountability Act (HIPAA), and privacy issues.

## EMS Staffing

When looking at EMS staffing, agencies do not only look at what the staffing needs are on the ambulance, but what other functions responders are being tasked with. EMS staffing is not simply the task of putting extra manpower or extra staffing out, it involves evaluating the issues that are causing the shortages and deciding how the organization needs to address them. Other issues with staffing are if there were two paramedics on an ambulance, when does it go to a one-paramedic, one-emergency medical technician (EMT) level? If an EMS agency is part of the fire service, will engines and trucks be taken out of service to put more people on the ambulance? Staffing the units may be difficult, as it must be done with the understanding that these other crews are going to lose possibly one third of their workforce

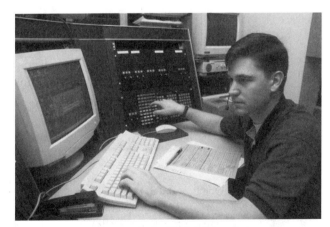

**Figure 12-2** EMS must coordinate with dispatchers during major disasters, so that telecommunicators may efficiently filter 9-1-1 calls.

should they choose to join the response effort. This may determine whether or not they will be able to respond.

## The Response Process

As incidents come up—whether they are bioterrorism, pandemic, SARS, or chemical attack responses—response processes are going to be altered. If a chemical weapon is deployed, the whole affected area of town may be secured, leaving responding units unable to enter. People may be bypassed because responding ambulances will not have the ability to get to the patients. The chemical may be pushed farther out due to winds or water.

Also, if there is an increase in ambulance calls and EMS is part of the fire service, does the agency take people off of engines and trucks to meet staffing needs? If the agency is a non-fire EMS agency, is there a plan in place directing EMS to ask the fire department: "Our call numbers have increased threefold. We need to come up with a modification. Is there a way, working together, that we can do this?" This allows EMS to know up front if there is a way that the agency can put additional staffing on the street in order to deal with the increased call volume. This can also help in dealing with increased acuity; depending on the types of patients present, they may be a higher acuity than what EMS are used to dealing with.

## Units in Service

Tied in with response are the units in service: If the EMS service normally operates 10 ambulances, does it need to go to 15? Is EMS capable of going up to 15? If the EMS system operates 10, and is forced to go down to five, what is the trigger mechanism to indicate that EMS needs to call for mutual aid? Those are the some of the basics that EMS needs to prepare for.

## Alternative Destinations

In considering large-scale incidents with a potential for a large surge of patients, EMS needs to work with the local hospitals to determine alternative destinations to deliver patients in case one hospital is overwhelmed. Depending on the incident, EMS may gain destinations or they may lose receiving facilities. Many states require EMS deliver only to emergency departments. If there is a disaster, however, an emergency department may be so overwhelmed that it may not be able to take patients such as those needing decontamination. The emergency department may also be overwhelmed with the amount of people showing up. If there is a plan in place, the question can be asked: "Under certain conditions, can we increase our destinations by allowing alternative treatment facilities to be opened?"

EMS needs to look not only at the destinations, but also at the transporting of people to destinations. Keeping in mind the trigger points to close a facility, when do EMS organizations put the call out for the need to open alternative treatment sites? It is important for EMS to plan for instances like this, and to coordinate planning so that it is done in a methodical process. This will enable everyone involved to be aware of what is happening. In addition to opening alternative treatment sites, EMS must also examine if there will be any alterations in standard of care, based on certain criteria. Furthermore, EMS needs to designate a person to determine

## Case Study

One hospital in the metropolitan Dallas area lost all communications in and out of the facility. There were no telecommunications capabilities, no one could call in, and no one could call out. EMS agencies transporting to that facility for stroke patients or patients that needed a catheterization were unable to get through; those patients were negatively impacted in terms of their level of care.

an alteration to standard of care. Agencies must ask: What are the trigger points or criteria? When will the start and the end points of the alteration to standard of care occur? These must be answered ahead of time.

There are three methods to define the trigger points for making alterations of care: "Option A" may be based on number of patients, "Option B" may be based on the number of calls over the base level of calls for that day or that month, and "Option C" may be based on the agent, once EMS actually knows what is going on. EMS should first determine the probability that an incident will happen, assess what will be a trigger factor, and then outline criteria to determine what deviation from standard procedure will need to be implemented. If EMS only has one set of circumstances to determine when to move up to alternative sites, this part of the plan may be inadequate.

An example could be a response for an anthrax incident: If a patient appears to have anthrax, that patient comes in and is treated promptly. If everyone is showing up with chemical burns, however, then the crews or treating responders will need to change their original plan for patient care to meet this new need. The triggers and resulting modifications to procedure must be well understood, based on the agent, staffing, or a number of different factors. For this reason, it is important that EMS coordinate this, based on an understanding of the incident conditions.

## Ambulance Capture

One of the things that EMS agencies need to examine is ambulance capture. This term refers to when ambulances arrive to the emergency department and are unable to return to service. In many urban areas this occurs often, as hospitals are filled to capacity and ambulances cannot off-load their patients. As facilities are increasing their intake of patients or experience an increase in the number of people flocking to them, any ambulances that are at the facility or en route to them will be captured or caught up in what is going on, so that they may be unable to clear the facility and be placed back in service. Responders have to plan on how to prevent ambulance capture as the incident evolves: Is there is a trigger point, what constitutes capture, and what will the agency do if this occurs? Is there an agreement in place with receiving facilities to expedite ambulance release? What number of captured ambulances constitutes a problem? What is the agency's plan if a significant number of units are captured; is there any plan for mutual aid or any other remedy?

## HIPAA and Privacy

The next issue EMS needs to consider is HIPAA and privacy. During a disaster or a public health emergency, HIPAA can be suspended. There has to be a start and an end point, however, if the EMS agency is going to alter their HIPAA precautions. EMS must ask: What specifically is going to be done to ensure patient privacy? They must look at what the plan of action is, and consider the involvement of medical control, hospital administrations, as well as state regulators. This will help identify what measures will ensure that patient privacy remains intact.

# Planning for Mass Disasters

When preplanning for a mass disaster, EMS must look at the potential impact on a community. Agencies need to assess the potential for a large-scale incident to overwhelm local and regional capabilities. They must analyze what is probable versus what is improbable (this goes back to the HVA). Gap analyses will enable EMS organizations to determine what shortfalls may occur.

EMS also needs to examine whether a given incident will require a standard or modified response: Will additional command personnel be needed? What kind of notification and activation is in place if initial standard response is inadequate? What are the trigger points for activation if the incident becomes larger in scope? There may be no changes; it may just be an observation and a report that could be a primary mission requiring some staff changes. A modified response may only involve adding one or two ambulances. Other things to consider as EMS responders pre-plan for disasters and pandemics include PPE, physical exams, or maybe putting one paramedic in a chase vehicle that goes to calls and triages patients ahead of the ambulance. It is important for EMS agencies to consider what needs to be done for a standard response, when each task will need to be accomplished, and what needs to be done once trigger points are reached that will change response procedure. These are key issues for EMS to consider to make sure responders have what they need to provide an effective emergency response.

## Selected References

Ammar, A: Role of leadership in disaster management and crowd control. *Prehosp Disaster Med* 2007;22(6):527–528.

Balicer, R, Omer, S, et al.: Local public health workers perceptions toward responding to an influenza pandemic. *BMC Public Health* 2006;6:99.

Barry, J: *The Great Influenza: The Story of the Deadliest Pandemic in History.* New York, NY: Penguin Books; 2005.

Bracha, HS, Burlke, F: Utility of fear severity and individual resilience scoring as a surge capacity, triage management tool during large scale bio-event disasters. *Prehosp Disaster Med* 2006;21(5):290–297.

Bremer, R: Policy development in disaster preparedness and management: Lessons learned from the January 2001 earthquake in Gujarat, India. *Prehosp Disaster Med* 2003;18(4):372–384.

Centers for Disease Control and Prevention: *In a Moment's Notice: Surge Capacity for Terrorist Bombings: Challenges and Proposed Solutions.* US Department of Health and Human Services; April, 2007.

Fisman, D: Dark clouds on the horizon: Preparing for the next influenza pandemic, part 1. *Medscape Infectious Diseases*; October, 2007.

Klein, K, Atlas, J, et al.: Testing emergency medical personnel response to patients with suspected infectious disease. *Prehosp Disaster Med* 2004;19(3):256–265.

Klein, K, Pepe, P, et al.: Evolving need for alternative triage management in public health emergencies: A Hurricane Katrina case study. *Disaster Med Public Health Prep* 2008;2(1):S40–S44.

Lettieri, C: Disaster medicine: Understanding the threat and minimizing the effects. *Medscape Emergency Medicine* 2006;1(1).

Loufty, M, Wallington, T, et al.: Hospital preparedness and SARS. *Emerging Infectious Diseases*, 2004;10(5). http://www.cdc.gov/ncidod/eid/index.htm.

Low, D. *SARS: Lessons from Toronto. Learning from SARS: Preparing for the Next Disease Outbreak* (Workshop Summary). Washington, D.C.: National Academy of Sciences; September 30-Oct 1, 2003.

NFPA 472. *Standard for Competence of Responders to Hazardous Materials/Weapons of Mass Destruction Incidents,* 2008 edition.

Noy, S: Minimizing casualties in biological and chemical threats (war and terrorism): The importance of information to the public in a prevention program. *Prehosp Disaster Med* 2004;19(1):29–36.

Phelps, S: Mission failure: Emergency medical services response to chemical, biological, radiological, nuclear, and explosive events. *Prehosp Disaster Med* 2007;22(4):293–296.

Silverman, A, Simor, A, et al.: Toronto emergency medical services and SARS [letter], in *Emerging Infectious Diseases* [serial on the Internet], 2004 Sept; 10(9).

United States Department of Homeland Security: Pandemic influenza preparedness: Alternate care site roles and responsibilities. *Lessons Learned Information Sharing.* https://www.llis.dhs.gov/index.do.

United States Department of Transportation: *Emergency Response Guidebook, 2008 edition.* Washington, D.C.: DOT; 2008.

Walz, B, Bissell, R, et al.: Vaccine administration by paramedics: A model for bioterrorism and disaster response preparation. *Prehosp Disaster Med* 2003;18(4):321–326.

Warrick, J: Crisis communications remain flawed. *The Washington Post.* December 10, 2005.

www.flu.gov. *The Next Flu Pandemic: What to Expect.* http://www.flu.gov/professional/community/nextflupandemic .html. Accessed December 1, 2009.

Bremer, R: Policy development in disaster preparedness and management: Lessons learned from the January 2001 earthquake in Gujarat, India. *Prehosp Disaster Med* 2003;18(4):372–384.

Buerhaus, P and Staiger, D: Trouble in the nurse labor market? Recent trends and future outlook. *Health Aff*, 1999;18(1):1, 214–222.

Calabro, J, Krohmer, J, et al.: *Provision of Emergency Medical Care for Crowds*. American College of Emergency Physicians EMS Committee; 1995–1996.

Cannon, MC: Task force smith: A study in (un)preparedness and (ir)responsibility. *Mil Rev*; 1988.

Carnevale, F, Alexander, E, et al.: Daily living with distress and enrichment: The moral experience of families with ventilator-assisted children at home. *Pediatrics* 2006;117(1):48–60.

Center for Catastrophe Preparedness and Response: *Emergency Medical Services: The Forgotten First Responder—A Report on the Critical Gaps in Organization and Deficits in Resources for America's Medical First Responders*. New York, NY: New York University; 2005.

Centers for Disease Control and Prevention: *Chemical Agents: Facts About Evacuation*. US Department of Health and Human Services; August 16, 2006.

Centers for Disease Control and Prevention: *Chemical Agents: Facts About Sheltering in Place*. US Department of Health and Human Services; August, 16, 2006.

Centers for Disease Control and Prevention: *In a Moment's Notice: Surge Capacity for Terrorist Bombings: Challenges and Proposed Solutions*. US Department of Health and Human Services; April, 2007.

Centers for Disease Control and Prevention: *The Public Health Response to Biological and Chemical Terrorism*. US Department of Health and Human Services; 2001.

Committee on Pediatric Emergency Medicine, Committee on Medical Liability, and the Task Force on Terrorism: The pediatrician and disaster preparedness. *Pediatrics* 2006;117(2):560–565.

Committee on the Future of Emergency Care in the United States Health System: *Hospital-Based Emergency Care: At the Breaking Point*. Washington, D.C.: The National Academies Press; 2007.

Committee to Identify Innovative Research Needs to Foster Improved Fire Safety in the United States, National Research Council: *Making the Nation Safe from Fire: A Path Forward in Research*. Washington, D.C.: The National Academies Press; 2003.

Congressional Charter of the American National Red Cross: *36 USC*; May, 2007.

Council on School Health: Disaster planning for schools. *Pediatrics* 2008;122(4):895–901.

Covey, SR: *Leadership: Great Leaders, Great Teams, Great Results*, audio CD. Salt Lake City, UT: Franklin Covey Company; 2007.

Cuny, F: Cuny memorial continuing education series, principles of disaster management: Lesson 1. *Prehosp Disaster Med* 1998;13(1):88–92.

Cuny, F: Cuny memorial continuing education series, principles of disaster management: Lesson 2. *Prehosp Disaster Med* 1998;13(2–4):63–79.

Davis, R: Only strong leaders can overhaul EMS. *USA Today*. May 20, 2005.

Deickmann. MD and Ronald, A: *Pediatric Education for Prehospital Professionals*. 2nd ed. Sudbury, MA: Jones and Bartlett Publishers; 2006.

Deitchman, S: What have we learned? Needs assessment. *Prehosp Disaster Med* 2005;20(6):468–470.

*Disaster Relief*, U.S. Code Title 42, chapter 68.

Doyle, CJ: Mass casualty incident. Integration with prehospital care. *Emergency Medicine Clinics of North America* 1990;8(1):163–175.

Drabek, T and Hoetmer, G: *Emergency Management: Principles and Practice for Local Government*. Washington, D.C.: International City/County Management Association; 1996.

Emergency Management Institute: Federal emergency management administration course IS-15.a, in *Special Events Contingency Planning for Public Safety Agencies*. http://training .fema.gov/EMIWeb/IS/IS15a.asp. Accessed December 1, 2009.

Emergency Medical Services Administrators Association of California: *Coordination of*

*Prehospital Emergency Services;* draft paper, undated.

*Emergency Planning and Community Right to Know Act (EPCRA),* U.S. Code Title 42, Chapter 116; October, 1986.

Emerson, N, Pesigan, A, et al.: First 30 days: Organizing rapid responses. *Prehosp Disaster Med* 2005;20(6):420–422.

*Federal Response to Hurricane Katrina: Lessons learned.* Washington, D.C.: The White House; February 23, 2006.

Feldman, M, Lukins, J, et al.: Half-a-million strong: The emergency medical services response to a single-day, mass-gathering event. *Prehosp Disaster Med* 2004;19(4):287–296.

*FEMA 592: Robert T. Stafford Disaster Relief and Emergency Assistance Act, as Amended, and Related Authorities;* Washington, D.C., FEMA; June, 2007.

FEMA: *Guide for All Hazards Planning Emergency Operations Planning.* Washington D.C.: FEMA; September, 1996.

FEMA: *Assistance to Firefighters Grant Program.* http://www.firegrantsupport.com. Accessed January 15, 2009.

Fernandez, LS, Byard, D,et al. : Frail elderly as disaster victims: Emergency management strategies. *Prehosp Disaster Med* 2002;17(2):67–74.

Fisman, D: Dark clouds on the horizon: Preparing for the next influenza pandemic, part 1. *Medscape Infectious Diseases;* October, 2007.

Flabouris, A, Nocera, A, et al.: Efficacy of critical incident monitoring for evaluating disaster medical readiness and response during the Sydney 2000 olympic games. *Prehosp Disaster Med* 2004;19(2):164–168.

Franco, C, Toner, E, et al.: The national disaster medical system: Past, present, and suggestions for the future. *Biosecurity and Bioterrorism* 2007;5:4,319–325.

Freyberg, C, Arquilla, B, et al.: Disaster preparedness: Hospital decontamination and the pediatric patient—Guidelines for hospitals and emergency planners. *Prehosp Disaster Med* 2008;23(2):166–172.

Gagliardi, M, Neighbors, M, et al.: Emergencies in the school setting: Are public school teachers adequately trained to respond? *Prehosp Disaster Med* 1994;9:222–225.

Gavagan, TF, Smart, K, et al.: Hurricane Katrina: Medical response at the Houston Astrodome/Reliant Center Complex. *South Med J* 2006;99(9):933–939.

George, ML: *Lean Six Sigma for Service.* New York, NY: The McGraw-Hill Companies; 2003.

Gershon, R, Qureshi, K, et al.: Factors associated with high-rise evacuation: Qualitative results from the World Trade Center evacuation study. *Prehosp Disaster Med* 2007;22(3):165–73.

Gildea, J and Etengoff, S: Vertical evacuation simulation of critically ill patients in a hospital. *Prehosp Disaster Med* 2005;20(4):243–248.

Goss, KC: Emergency management & special events: Challenges, support, best practices. *DomPrep Journal* 2004;5:12–13.

Graham, J, Shirm, S, et al.: Mass casualty events at schools: A national preparedness survey. *Pediatrics* 2006;117(1):e8–e15.

Grange, JT: Planning for large events. *Current Sports Medicine Reports.* 2002;1(3):156–161.

Grange, JT, Baumann, GW, et al.: On-site physicians reduce ambulance transports at mass gatherings. *Prehosp Emerg Care* 2003;7:322–326.

Grentenkort, P, Harke, H, et al.: Interface between hospital and fire authorities: A concept for management of incidents in hospitals. *Prehosp Disaster Med* 2002;17(1):42–47.

Hamilton, DR, Gavagan, TF, et al.: Houston's medical disaster response to Hurricane Katrina: Part 1, The initial medical response from trauma service area Q. *Ann Emerg Med* 2009;53(4):505–514.

Hamilton, DR, Gavagan, TF, et al.: Houston's medical disaster response to Hurricane Katrina: Part 2, transitioning from emergency evacuee care to community health care. *Ann Emerg Med* 2009;53(4):515–527.

Hazinski, M, Markensen, D, et al. and the American Heart Association: Response to cardiac arrest and selected life-threatening medical emergencies: The medical emergency response plan for schools. *Circulation* 2004;109(2):278–291.

Hersche, B and Wenker, O: Principles of hospital disaster planning. *The Internet Journal of Rescue and Disaster Medicine* 2003; 1(2).

Hooke, W and Rodgers, P, eds.: *Public Health Risks of Disasters: Communication, Infrastructure and Preparedness.* Washington, D.C.: The National Academies Press; 2005.

Howe, E, Victor, D, et al.: Chief complaints, diagnoses, and medications prescribed seven weeks post-Katrina in New Orleans. *Prehosp Disaster Med* 2008;23(1):41–47.

Hsu, EB, Jenckes, MW, et al.: *Training of Hospital Staff to Respond To A Mass Casualty Incident. Evidence Report/Technology Assessment: Number 95.* Rockville, MD: Agency for Healthcare Research and Quality; April, 2004.

Hsu, E, Grabowski, J, et al.: Effects of local emergency departments of large scale urban chemical fire with hazardous materials spill. *Prehosp Disaster Med* 2002;17(4):196–201.

Hsu, E, Jenckes, M, et al.: Effectiveness of hospital staff mass-casualty incident training methods: A systematic literature review. *Prehosp Disaster Med* 2004;19(3):191–199.

Hutton, DW: *The Change Agent's Handbook.* Milwaukee, WI: ASQ Quality Press; 1994.

International Association of Fire Fighters and International Association of Fire Chiefs: *Everyone Comes Home Initiative.* http://www.everyonegoeshome.com. Accessed January 16, 2009.

International City/County Management Association: *Managing Fire and Rescue Services.* Washington, D.C.: ICMA Press; 2002.

International City/County Management Association: *Managing Fire Services,* 2nd ed. Washington, D.C.: ICMA Press; 1988.

International Kickboxing Federation: *Event Medical Staff Information and Requirements.* http://www.ikfkickboxing.com/Physicians.htm. Accessed December 1, 2009.

Jasolow, D, Yancey II, A, et al.: *Mass Gathering Medical Care: The Medical Director's Checklist.* Lenexa, KS: National Association of EMS Physicians; 2000.

Johnston, C and Redlener, I: Critical concepts for children in disasters identified by hands-on professionals: Summary of issues demanding solutions before the next one. *Pediatrics* 2006;117(5):S458–S460.

Joint Commission on Accreditation of Healthcare Organizations: *Standing Together: An Emergency Planning Guide for America's Communities.* Washington, D.C.: JCAHO; 2005.

Jolly, BT and Martinez, R: Heart stopping action: Whether it's a sporting event or rock concert, medical emergencies can spoil the fun and create liability unless management plans ahead. *Security Management;* April, 2004.

Kanawha Putnam Emergency Planning Committee: *Kanawha Putnam Emergency Management Plan* (Annex A04, "Evacuation"). Charlestown, WV; 2006.

Kano, M, Ramirez, M, et al.: Are schools prepared for emergencies: A baseline assessment of emergency preparedness at school sites in three Los Angeles County school districts. *Educ Urban Soc* 2007;39:3399–3422.

Kanter, R, Andrake, J, et al.: Developing consensus on appropriate standards of disaster care for children. *Disaster Med Public Health Prep* 2009;3(1):5–7.

Kerins, D and Cortacans, HP: *Pre-Planning and Preparedness Pay Off; New Jersey EMS Response to US Airways Hudson River Crash.* http://www.JEMS.com. Accessed February 2, 2009.

Klein, K, Atlas, J, et al.: Testing emergency medical personnel response to patients with suspected infectious disease. *Prehosp Disaster Med* 2004;19(3):256–265.

Klein, K, Pepe, P, et al.: Evolving need for alternative triage management in public health emergencies: A Hurricane Katrina case study. *Disaster Med Public Health Prep* 2008; 2(1):S40–S44.

Knouss, RF: National disaster medical system. *Public Health Reports,* supplement 2, volume 116. Rockville, MD: US Department of Heath and Human Services, Office of Emergency Preparedness/Federal Emergency Management Agency; 2001.

Kramer, WM and Bahme, CW: *Fire Officer's Guide to Disaster Control.* 2nd ed. Saddle Brook, NJ: Fire Engineering Books and Videos, Penwell Publishing; 1992.

Krebs, D: EMS preplanning for large public events. *Fire Eng*; June, 2001.

Kuba, M, Dorian, A, et al.: *Elderly Populations in Disasters: Recounting Evacuation Processes from Two Skilled-Care Facilities in Florida*, UCLA Center for Public Health and Disasters; August, 2004.

Laditka, SB, Laditka, JN, et al.: Disaster preparedness for vulnerable persons receiving in-home, long-term care in South Carolina. *Prehosp Disaster Med* 2008;23(2):133–142.

Landesman, LY: *Public Health Management of Disasters: The Practice Guide*. 2nd ed. Washington, D.C.: American Public Health Association; 2005.

Leonard, RB, Winslow, JE, et al.: Planning medical care for high-risk mass gatherings. *Internet Journal of Rescue and Disaster Medicine* 2007;6(1).

Lettieri, C: Disaster medicine: Understanding the threat and minimizing the effects. *Medscape Emergency Medicine* 2006;1(1).

Levinson, DR *Nursing Home Emergency Preparedness and Response During Recent Hurricanes*. Washington, D.C.: Department of Health and Human Services, Office of Inspector General; August, 2006.

Lintu, N, Health, M, et al.: Reactions to cold exposure emphasize the need for weather protection in prehospital care: An experimental study. *Prehosp Disaster Med* 2006;21(5):316–320.

Loufty, M, Wallington, T, et al.: Hospital preparedness and SARS. *Emerging Infectious Diseases*, 2004;10(5). http://www.cdc.gov/ncidod/eid/index.htm.

Low, D. *SARS: Lessons from Toronto. Learning from SARS: Preparing for the Next Disease Outbreak* (Workshop Summary). Washington, D.C.: National Academy of Sciences; September 30-Oct 1, 2003.

Lukins, JL, Feldman MJ, et al.: A paramedic-staffed rehydration unit at a mass gathering. *Prehosp Emerg Care* 2004;8(4):411–416.

Ma, OJ, Millward, L, et al.: EMS medical coverage at PGA tour events. *Prehosp Emerg Care* 2002;6(1):11–14.

Maguire, B, Dean, S, et al.: Epidemic and bioterrorism preparation among emergency medical services systems. *Prehosp Disaster Med* 2007;22(3):237–242.

Manning, F and Goldfrank, L, ed.: *Preparing for Terrorism: Tools for Evaluating the Metropolitan Medical Response System Program*. Committee on Evaluation of the Metropolitan Medical Response System, Board on Health Sciences Policy. Washington, D.C.: The National Academies Press; 2002.

Markenson, D, Reynolds, S, and Committee on Pediatric Emergency Medicine and Task Force on Terrorism: The pediatrician and disaster preparedness. *Pediatrics* 2006;117(2):340–362.

McGovern, JE: Casualty evacuation and patient movement. *Special Operations Medical Support*. Lenexa, KS: National Association of Emergency Physicians; 2009.

Merriam-Webster Collegiate Dictionary. Springfield, MA: Merriam-Webster; 1961.

Mignone, T and Davidson, R: Public health response actions and the use of emergency operations centers. *Prehosp Disaster Med* 2003;18(3):217–218.

Miller, AC and Arquilla, B: Chronic diseases and natural hazards: Impact of disasters on diabetic, renal, and cardiac patients. *Prehosp Disaster Med* 2008;23(3):185–194.

Milsten, AM: *From Start to Finish: Physician Usefulness at Mass Gathering Event*. American College of Emergency Physicians; 2009. http:// www.acep.org/ACEPmembership.

Milsten, A, Maguire, B, et al.: Mass-gathering medical care: A review of the literature. *Prehosp Disaster Med* 2002;17(3):151–162.

Milsten, A, Seaman, K, et al.: Variables influencing medical usage rates, injury patterns, and levels of care for mass gatherings. *Prehosp Disaster Med* 2003;18(4):334–346.

Mohammed, A, Mann, H, et al.: Impact of London's terrorist attacks on a major trauma center in London. *Prehosp Disaster Med* 2006;21(5):340–344.

Moles, TM: Emergency medical services systems and HAZMAT major incidents. *Resuscitation* 1999;42(2):103–116.

Morimura, N, Katsumi, A, et al.: Analysis of patient load data from the 2002 FIFA World

Cup Korea/Japan. *Prehosp Disaster Med* 2004;19(3):278–284.

National Association of Emergency Managers: *Emergency Management Assistance Compact Overview*. Lexington, KY. http://www.nemaweb.org. Accessed December 1, 2009.

National Disaster Medical System (NDMS): *Federal Coordinating Center Guide*. Washington, D.C.: Department of Health and Human Services; 2006.

National Fire Protection Association: *Learn Not to Burn*. (A copyrighted curriculum for young children first implemented by the NFPA in 1978 and now in its third edition, part of the curriculum in more than 40,000 schools.) Quincy, MA: NFPA; 1978.

National Response Team Response Subcommittee Workgroup: *Joint Information Center Model: Collaborative Communications During Emergency Response*. Washington, D.C.: The National Response Team; 2000.

NFPA 472. *Standard for Competence of Responders to Hazardous Materials/Weapons of Mass Destruction Incidents*, 2008 edition.

Noji, EK, ed. *The Public Health Consequences of Disasters*. New York, NY: Oxford University Press; 1997.

North Carolina Division of Emergency Management, North Carolina Division of Public Health, North Carolina Office of Emergency Medical Services: *Hurricane Katrina After Action Review and Recommendations*. Emergency Support Function 8 Health and Medical, State of Mississippi; June 1, 2006.

Noy, S: Minimizing casualties in biological and chemical threats (war and terrorism): The importance of information to the public in a prevention program. *Prehosp Disaster Med* 2004;19(1):29–36.

O'Sullivan, T, Amaratunga, C, et al.: If schools are closed, who will watch our kids? Family caregiving and other sources of role conflict among nurses during large scale outbreaks. *Prehosp Disaster Med* 2009;24(4):321–325.

Occupational Health and Safety Administration. *Hazard Communication Standard*. 29 CFR 1910.1200.

Olness, K, Mandalakas, A, et al.: The children in disasters project: Addressing the special needs of children in man-made and natural disasters. *Pediatrics* 2008;121;S115.

Olympia, R, Wan, E, et al.: The preparedness of schools to respond to emergencies in children: A national survey of school nurses. *Pediatrics* 2005;116(6):e738–e745.

Pan-American Health Organization, Regional Office, World Health Organization: *Hospitals in Disasters: Handle with Care Discussion Guide*; July, 2003.

Pennsylvania Emergency Management Agency: *Special Event Emergency Action Plan Guide*. Harrisburg, PA: Pennsylvania Emergency Management Agency. http://www.portal.state.pa.us. Accessed December 1, 2009.

Phelps, S: Mission failure: Emergency medical services response to chemical, biological, radiological, nuclear, and explosive events. *Prehosp Disaster Med* 2007;22(4):293–296.

Pirrallo, RG and Cady, CE: Lessons learned from an emergency medical services fire safety intervention. *Prehosp Emerg Care* 2004;8(2):171–174.

Regional Office for South East Asia World Health Organization: Regional meeting on health aspects of disaster preparedness and response. *Prehosp Disaster Med* 2006;21(5):s62–s78.

Reijneveld, S: Psychosocial implications of disaster on children and pediatric care. *Pediatrics* 2006;117(5):1865–1866.

Rowitz, L: *Public Health for the 21st Century: The Prepared Leader*. Sudbury, MA: Jones and Bartlett Publishers; 2006.

Rubin, J: *Recurring Pitfalls in Hospital Preparedness and Response*. http://www.homelandsecurity.org; January, 2004. Accessed August 28, 2007.

Salhanick, S, Shehan, W, et al.: Use and analysis of field triage criteria for mass gathering. *Prehosp Disaster Med* 2003;18(4):347–352.

Sanderson, P: Liability involving special events, in *New Hampshire Town & City*. Concord, NH: New Hampshire Local Government Center; May, 2009.

Schulte, D and Meade, DM: The Papal chase. The Pope's visit: A 'mass' gathering. *Emerg Med Services* 1993;22(1):46–49,65–75,79.

Schultz, C, Koenig, K, et al.: Benchmarking for hospital evacuation: A critical data collection tool. *Prehosp Disaster Med* 2005;20(5):331–342.

Select Bipartisan Committee to Investigate the Preparation for and Response to Hurricane Katrina: *A Failure of Initiative Final Report of the Select Bipartisan Committee to Investigate the Preparation for and Response to Hurricane Katrina.* February, 2006.

Silverman, A, Simor, A, et al.: Toronto emergency medical services and SARS [letter], in *Emerging Infectious Diseases* [serial on the Internet], 2004 Sept; 10(9).

Smilde-van den Doel, D, Smit, C, et al.: School performance and social-emotional behavior of primary school children before and after a disaster. *Pediatrics* 2006;118(5):e1311–1320.

Smith, JP *Strategic and Tactical Considerations on the Fireground.* Upper Saddle River, NJ: Brady Books, Pearson; 2002.

Snowden, L and Kyle, L S: Crowds, cold challenge D.C. responders at inauguration. *EMSResponder.com*; January 20, 2009.

Snowden, L and Kyle, LS: Inaugural response: An inside look. *EMSResponder.com*; January 18, 2009.

State of California. *California Emergency Services Act,* definition, section 8558(a).

State of Missouri, State Emergency Management Agency: NIMS definitions and acronyms. http://sema.dps.mo.gov/Planning/NIMS%20Definitions.doc. Accessed December 1, 2009.

State of Texas Emergency Management, Governor's Division of Emergency Management: *2007 Hurricane Dean After Action Report*; November 26, 2007.

Stenberg, E, Lee, G, et al.: Counting crises: US hospital evacuations 1971–1999. *Prehosp Disaster Med* 2004;19(2):150–157.

Taaffee, K, Kohl, R, et al.: *Hospital Evacuation: Issues and Complexities Proceeding of the 2005 Winter Simulation Conference.* Clemson, SC: Clemson University; 2005.

*The Drug Free Schools and Communities Act Amendments,* Public Law 101-226,103 Stat. 1928; December 12, 1989.

The IEMS National Advisory Committee: Chief executive officer's checklist. *The CEO's Disaster Survival Kit.* Federal Emergency Management Agency and the United States Fire Administration; 1988.

Thierbach, A, Wolcke, B, et al.: Medical support for children's mass gatherings. *Prehosp Disaster Med* 2003;18(1):14–19.

Thorne, C, Levitin, H, et al.: A pilot assessment of hospital preparedness for bioterrorism events. *Prehosp Disaster Med* 2006;21(6):414–422.

Tokuda, Y, Kikuchi, M, et al.: Pre-hospital management of sarin nerve gas terrorism in urban settings: 10 years of progress after the Tokyo subway sarin attack. *Resuscitation* 2006;68(2):193–202.

Treat, K, Williams, J, et al.: Hospital preparedness for weapons of mass destruction incidents: An initial assessment. *Ann Emerg Med* 2001; 38(5):562–565.

United States Department of Defense: *Dictionary of Military and Associated Terms.* Joint Publication 1-02. April 12, 2001 (as amended through March 17, 2009).

United States Department of Homeland Security: *Department of Homeland Security Spending Documents 2007.* http://www.dhs.gov. Accessed December 30, 2008.

United States Department of Homeland Security: Incident management: Alerting hospitals in close proximity to a mass casualty incident. *Lessons Learned Information Sharing.* https://www.llis.dhs.gov/index.do.

United States Department of Homeland Security: Mass evacuation: Developing a contraflow plan. *Lessons Learned Information Sharing.* https://www.llis.dhs.gov/index.do.

United States Department of Homeland Security: Mass evacuation: Triage units at embarkation points. *Lessons Learned Information Sharing.* https://www.llis.dhs.gov/index.do.

United States Department of Homeland Security: Pandemic influenza preparedness: Alternate care site roles and responsibilities. *Lessons Learned Information Sharing.* https://www.llis.dhs.gov/index.do.

United States Department of Homeland Security: Shelter operations: Establishing a quiet room to calm residents with mental illness. *Lessons Learned Information Sharing.* https://www.llis.dhs.gov/index.do.

United States Department of Homeland Security: *National Response Framework*; January 2008. http://www.dhs.gov/files/programs/editorial_0566.shtm. Accessed December 1, 2009.

United States Department of Transportation: *Emergency Response Guidebook, 2008 edition.* Washington, D.C.: DOT; 2008.

United States Department of Transportation: *Traffic Safety Facts 2006: A Compilation of Motor Vehicle Crash Data from the Fatality Analysis Reporting System and the General Estimates System.* Washington, D.C.: DOT, National Center for Statistics and Analysis; 2006.

United States Department of Transportation: Managing travel for planned special events, in *Publication No: FHWA-NHI-03-120.* Washington, D.C.: DOT; 2003. http:// www .ops.fhwa.dot.gov/publications. Accessed December 1, 2009.

United States Fire Administration. *FA-166 Risk Management Practices in the Fire Service.* Emmitsburg, MD: USFA; December, 1996.

United States Fire Administration: Topical fire research series. *Medical Facility Fires* 2002; 2(8).

United States Fire Administration: Fire safety lasts a lifetime: A fire safety factsheet for older adults and their caregivers; Emmitsburg, MD: USFA; March, 2006.

United States Fire Administration, Federal Emergency Management Agency, Department of Homeland Security. *The National Fire Incident Reporting System (NFIRS).* Emmitsburg, MD: USFA.

United States National Commission on Fire Prevention and Control: *America Burning: The Report of the National Commission on Fire Prevention and Control*; 1973.

United States National Committee for the Decade for Natural Disaster Reduction: *A Safer Future: Reducing the Impacts of Natural Disasters.* National Research Council; 1991.

Vilke, G, Smith, A, et al.: Impact of the San Diego county firestorm on emergency medical services. *Prehosp Disaster Med* 2006;21(5):353–358.

Waldman, R: What have we learned? Filling gaps in available services. *Prehosp Disaster Med* 2005;20(6):475–479.

Walz, B, Bissell, R, et al.: Vaccine administration by paramedics: A model for bioterrorism and disaster response preparation. *Prehosp Disaster Med* 2003;18(4):321–326.

Warrick, J: Crisis communications remain flawed. *The Washington Post.* December 10, 2005.

Winslow, JE and Goldstein, AO: Spectator risks at sporting events. *The Internet Journal of Law, Healthcare and Ethics* 2007;4:2.

World Health Organization: *Studies on ED Planning and Hazards.* http://www.who.int. Accessed February 2, 2009.

www.flu.gov. *The Next Flu Pandemic: What to Expect.* http://www.flu.gov/professional/community/nextflupandemic.html. Accessed December 1, 2009.

Zane, R and Prestipino, A: Implementing the hospital emergency incident command system: An integrated delivery system's experience. *Prehosp Disaster Med* 2004;19(4):311–317.